Contents

About the authors

Donna Brayford is a community midwife and teenage pregnancy link midwife at the University Hospital of North Staffordshire. She has a passion to deliver high standards of care as a midwife and help others to practise in clinically effective ways.

Ruth Chambers has been a general practitioner for more than 20 years. She is currently a GP, a clinical lead for the Royal College of General Practitioners and Professor of Primary Care Development at Staffordshire University. Her interest in clinical effectiveness and clinical audit grew from her three-year spell as Chairman of Staffordshire Medical Audit Advisory Group in the 1990s.

Ruth has run several series of clinical effectiveness and clinical governance workshops, teaching a mix of primary and community care health professionals clinical effectiveness skills in easy steps and an understanding of clinical governance. The experiences of those workshops have informed this book.

Elizabeth Boath is a Reader in Health and Social Care and a Learning and Teaching Fellow at Staffordshire University. Liz had a special interest in the field of perinatal mental health. Her interest in clinical effectiveness and clinical governance emerged from her time as a research facilitator, during which she facilitated and taught on the series of workshops used to develop this book.

David Rogers is the clinical effectiveness librarian for the Bedside Clinical Guidelines Partnership. He has taught thousands of health professionals how to seek for the evidence base for their practice over the years. David also provides the evidence for clinical guidelines used by 25 hospital trusts across the Midlands and beyond.

Preface

The best practice discussed in this book is not easily achieved in the current climate of our maternity health system. Midwives can be undermined by limitations and constraints in financial resources, coping with daily increasing workloads. Midwives may lack the time to actively participate in, conduct and implement research, and to find and critically evaluate evidence which they can use in their everyday practice. In some trusts there may be an inadequate facility for personal and professional development, with study leave and funding regularly cancelled due to staff shortages. This then restricts midwives' practice, to allow them to implement changes based on evidence. But, despite these organisational pressures, we as midwives must be dedicated to providing safe care for individual women and their babies, and moving maternity care forward.

Hopefully the learning and strategies covered in this book will assist you in bringing your everyday work up to the high standards of care that match evidence-based best practice, and getting ready for revalidation. As you do so you should document the standards of your everyday work so that you can demonstrate that you are competent and performing well at your annual appraisals. Then it will be a small step to produce evidence of your midwifery practice for the revalidation of your professional qualifications in the near future.

Donna Brayford
Community midwife
January 2008

Introduction

Clinical effectiveness and clinical governance are about knowing what you should be doing and being able to put that knowledge into midwifery practice

Overall aim of the programme

To increase awareness of, and skills in, the adoption of an evidence-based approach to the practice and delivery of healthcare.

Objectives of this book

This programme is for all midwives to learn how to:

- ask the right question – it must be important to you and your colleagues
- look for the evidence and do a literature search
- receive and incorporate constructive criticism from colleagues about their developing questions and search for evidence
- select the best evidence – what to do where no strong evidence exists
- evaluate and interpret the evidence, such as read and extract information from a report
- apply the evidence as appropriate in a practice, unit or department
- act on the evidence to improve the practice of clinical effectiveness
- promote a culture of clinical governance.

Self-assessment of where you are now with clinical effectiveness and clinical governance

Before you start working through the clinical effectiveness and clinical governance programme, assess your baseline knowledge and attitudes. You should complete a similar self-assessment when you have worked through the book, so that you can compare your answers to see how your knowledge and skills have increased. Please circle as many answers as apply, or fill in the information requested.

1 How confident do you feel that you are capable of practising clinical effectiveness to be able to:

ask a relevant question?	*Very*	*Somewhat*	*Not at all*
undertake a search of the literature?	*Very*	*Somewhat*	*Not at all*
find readily available evidence?	*Very*	*Somewhat*	*Not at all*
weigh up available evidence?	*Very*	*Somewhat*	*Not at all*
decide if changes in practice are warranted?	*Very*	*Somewhat*	*Not at all*
make changes in practice as appropriate?	*Very*	*Somewhat*	*Not at all*

2 Have you ever searched the literature yourself for an answer
to a question?   *Yes/No*

If '*Yes*':

•   which database(s) have you used?

Medline   Cochrane   OMNI   Other (what?)

•   where did you search the literature?

Medical library   At work   At home   Other (where?)

•   did you have any help in searching the literature?

None   Healthcare librarian   Friend/family   Work colleague   Other (who?)

3 Have you ever asked someone else to search the literature for you? *Yes/No*

If '*Yes*':

•   who did the search for you?
•   why didn't you do the search yourself?

*Lack of time   Lack of skill   Lack of access   Other reason
                                   to databases*

4 Can you complete the following list from your own knowledge, describing
the features of different types or levels of evidence in decreasing order of
robustness from very strong evidence to none at all?

Type	Features
I	Strong evidence from at least one systematic review of multiple, well-designed, randomised controlled trials
II	
III	
IV	
V	Opinions of respected authorities, descriptive studies, reports of experts

5 If you have previously searched for the evidence to answer a question you
had posed, what did you do with the result of your search? (Circle all that apply.)

- *Discussed it with colleagues at work*
- *Discussed it with friends or family*
- *Made change(s) to an aspect of work*
- *Decided against making any change(s) to any aspect of work*
- *Other outcome – what?*

6 To what extent is evidence-based healthcare central to your own practice?
(Circle all that apply.)

- *I have no idea whether my everyday practice is evidence-based most of the time*
- *I assume that my everyday practice is evidence-based whenever possible, but I've no evidence for that assumption*
- *I ensure that my everyday practice is evidence-based by regularly comparing my practice against published standards of best practice and making appropriate changes*

7 How many of these principles of good practice in clinical governance do you
generally include as part of your quality improvement work? (Circle all that
apply.)

- *I actively promote or participate in multidisciplinary working*
- *I address national, local, organisational or professional priorities in my work*
- *I try to achieve partnership working, e.g. between agencies, between management/clinicians*
- *I incorporate input from patients in my work (e.g. users, carers, the public) in training, planning, monitoring or delivery of healthcare*
- *I look for potential to achieve health gains in the way I organise my work*
- *My everyday work is based on evidence-based practice, policy or management*
- *I can demonstrate the standards of care or services that I or my team achieve*

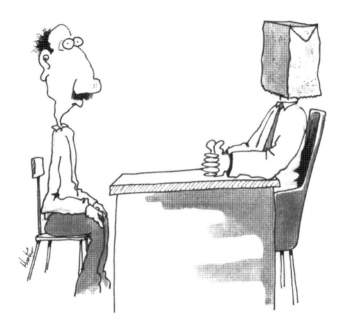

**Find out how to practise clinical effectiveness – don't shut your eyes
to the changes going on around you.**

What are clinical effectiveness and evidence-based healthcare?

Clinical effectiveness is 'the extent to which specific clinical interventions, when deployed in the field for a particular patient or population, do what they are intended to do – i.e. maintain and improve health and secure the greatest possible health gain from the available resources. To be reasonably certain that an intervention has produced health benefits, it needs to be shown to be capable of producing worthwhile benefit (efficacy and cost-effectiveness) and that it has produced that benefit in practice'.[1]

Evidence-based healthcare 'takes place when decisions that affect the care of patients are taken with due weight accorded to all valid, relevant information'.[2]

Evidence-based healthcare is the 'conscientious, explicit, and judicious use of current best evidence in making decisions about the care of individual patients. The practice of evidence-based medicine means integrating individual clinical expertise with the best available external clinical evidence from systematic research'.[3]

A problem-solving approach based on good evidence can also be applied to non-clinical decision making, such as most areas of management and resource allocation, as well as to clinical situations.

The three components of best possible clinical decision making[4,5] are *clinical expertise, patient preferences* and *clinical research evidence*. Clinical expertise and patient preferences may override the research evidence in some situations and for some patients. For example, patients may opt for less invasive treatment, or a sick patient may be too frail to undergo treatment with significant side effects.

Clinical audit remains an important tool for determining whether actual performance compares with evidence-based standards and, if not, what changes are needed to improve performance. Clinical audit is 'the systematic and critical analysis of the quality of clinical care, including the procedures used for diagnosis, treatment and care, the associated use of resources and the resulting outcome and quality of life for the patient'.[1] In other words, clinical audit helps you to reach a standard of clinical work as near to best practice as possible.

The process of achieving evidence-based healthcare can be divided into four sections:

1 the composition of a good question
2 a search of the literature to find the 'best' evidence available
3 an evaluation of what seems to be the most appropriate and relevant literature
4 the application of the evidence or findings.

What is the evidence for evidence-based healthcare?

There is growing evidence for the implementation of evidence-based healthcare.[6] Promoting Action on Clinical Effectiveness (PACE), a King's Fund programme, developed evidence-based practice as a routine way of working for health services. An interim report[6] described the successful outcomes when clinical effectiveness was linked to local needs and priorities so long as clinicians, managers, policy makers and patients were all involved in the process.

Practising in an evidence-based way:

- will promote your job satisfaction and feeling of being in control over your work
- can be used to justify maintaining or increasing budget allocations to particular areas of work
- will enhance your capability to do what's best for the patient.[7]

Why midwives need information

Midwives need to be well informed to be able to advise and inform patients appropriately. Patients who access the Internet and other electronic databases are starting to use that information to challenge clinicians' decisions about their care.

Clinicians will come under more pressure to respond to patients who have easy access to detailed information obtained from various sources, some of which will be inaccurate and misleading. The movement to patient empowerment has been generally welcomed, but may be threatening for clinicians who are insufficiently prepared to talk to well-informed patients, because they are unsure of their own knowledge base, time pressured, or do not understand how to assess what is the best evidence.

Clinicians will need to develop skills in finding and judging medical information, and communicating such information to patients appropriately. Health professionals may lay themselves open to complaints or legal procedures if they fail to adopt best practice through ignorance of the available evidence. Clinicians need good communication skills as well as reliable information when advising patients.

Patients are increasingly encouraged to seek out information from the Internet themselves. Midwives can help patients by indicating which electronic sources are most likely to be appropriate and reliable.

Ultimately, reliable and accurate information, good communication skills and patient empowerment are all features of a good quality primary healthcare service and a positive culture of clinical governance. Midwives and managers need good information when assessing the health needs of their patient populations, commissioning healthcare services and striving to reduce inequalities. Detailed information is needed to distinguish between different subgroups of the population, between patient populations and others elsewhere, or to monitor variations in performance between different practitioners and general practices or hospitals.

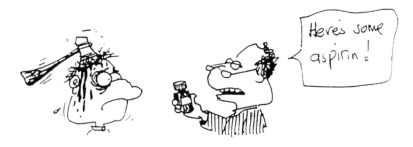

Quality of care may be compromised ...

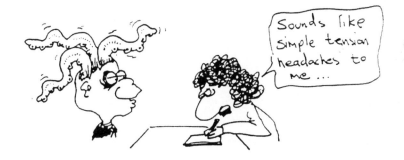

without clinical effectiveness

Are midwives ready for evidence-based healthcare?

With the creation of specialist and consultant roles for midwives and a change to degree level training, midwives have developed a more positive attitude towards research-based practice.[7] But these attitudes have not necessarily led to effective implementation of evidence in practice. Relatively few midwives actually make significant use of evidence to advance their practice.

Midwives are dedicated to the improvement of health of women, and the reduction of adverse health outcomes. Understanding evidence-based research plays a critical role in achieving these goals. A survey of researchers suggested that for midwives to understand evidence-based healthcare they do not need the skills to do research, but they must be able to understand and interpret published research, and differentiate the good from the bad research report.[8]

Researchers were asked about their main concerns regarding evidence-based practice, particularly in relation to midwifery. They expressed concern that there can be a strong emphasis on making autonomous decisions on the basis of personal history, professional tradition and personal skills, rather than evidence-based research.[8] Midwives can feel alienated by quantitative research design and because so few research trials involve midwives themselves.[8] Persistent barriers to carrying out and applying research in respect of midwifery practice include organisational issues, lack of a research culture, changing attitudes, lack of knowledge, skills and confidence, poor access to research and discomfort with information technology.[9]

Other adverse comments about evidence-based practice include fear of the imposition of too rigid a healthcare culture, the loss of an overriding duty to provide compassionate and sensitive care[10] and that wholesale evidence-based practice is unrealistic because it is not affordable. Some people mistrust the research–evidence base component of evidence-based practice because of the unreliability of some of the published literature; study biases are not always sufficiently recognised or acknowledged and, in occasional cases, have been discredited by sensational scandals involving researchers falsifying data.

Putting evidence into practice is a long and complicated process. Research from the King's Fund and others has emphasised that success in applying evidence-based practice is more likely: if there are sufficient resources (time, money and skills); if the proposed changes offer benefits to frontline staff; if the right people are 'signed up' to the proposed changes early enough; if the change is managed in an interactive way; and if research underpinning the change is clearly related to practice.[11] Many different approaches are being tried to overcome practitioners' and managers' seeming reluctance to change their practice according to new evidence as research is published. Governments are translating their policies into practical guidance and toolkits for implementing national standards or frameworks.[12,13] But we have a long way to go before the policies that governments evolve are evidence-based themselves.[14]

Learning by portfolio

Portfolio-based learning has been promoted since the early 1990s as a style of education that allows individuals to progress at their own pace. People can adopt education relevant to their needs, and composing a portfolio allows plenty of opportunities for reflection. Portfolio-based learning is not an easy option[15] compared to relatively passive types of learning such as listening to lectures. It takes a great deal of effort to complete a successful portfolio built on your past experiences and to progress through the stages of gathering and processing new information, critical reflection, interpretation and application. But it is worth it. The satisfaction that comes from completing a portfolio is as much about being in control of your own education as acquiring new knowledge, attitudes and/or skills.[16,17]

Another advantage of composing a portfolio is that on-the-job learning is relevant to your work and life, and this is likely to retain your interest. At the end of the project you will have discovered that you have further educational and developmental needs. And hopefully you will be discussing these within your annual appraisal. You will then have to decide whether or not you have taken learning about this topic, i.e. how to practise clinical effectiveness, as far as your resources (time, cost and effort) permit.

So, using a portfolio-based approach to acquire the basic ability to practise clinical effectiveness, you should aim in your work programme to:

- identify the learning task(s), e.g. what capability you need to be able to practise clinical effectiveness and clinical governance
- set learning goals, e.g. learn to frame a question; search for, interpret and apply the evidence
- identify ways of achieving your goals by, for example, working through this book, peer group discussion, visiting colleagues, undertaking a (supervised) literature search, exploring the Internet, reading more widely, making changes at work. Use this information to compose your personal development plan
- identify learning resources, e.g. electronic databases in the healthcare library, the Internet, books, journals, video tuition tapes, local courses, correspondence from hospital specialists
- monitor how well the learning is going, e.g. reflect on the development of your knowledge and skills, seek a colleague's view of your work. Work with others in your practice or at the trust to feed your learning needs into the workplace development plan
- list your achievements, e.g. run through a cycle of clinical effectiveness
- use what you have learned, e.g. make change(s) at work as a result of obtaining evidence or new information as part of clinical governance.

Some people prefer to work alone, while others find that having a mentor to help build the portfolio is useful. A mentor can help you to determine your learning needs, develop a study plan, support and challenge the work done, identify further learning gaps and generally help you to stay on course. To some extent the way that this clinical effectiveness learning programme is set out obviates the need for a mentor, but if you think a mentor might facilitate your work, consider asking your line manager or local tutor to recommend a mentor; or maybe a colleague could work alongside you sharing the 'programme' too, as a 'co-mentor' or 'buddy'.[15]

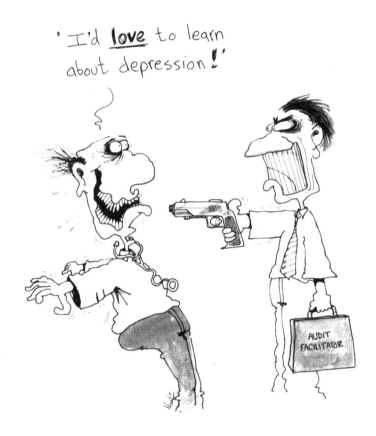

Clinical effectiveness requires real commitment.

Electronic databases

The Internet

The Internet is the largest computer network in the world to which almost any type of computer can link. Most academic institutions are connected to the Joint Academic Network (JANET) and its Internet service (JIPS); staff and students can then access the Internet free on campus, or can dial up from home via a modem for the cost of a local phone call. NHSNet is the equivalent for all NHSstaff.

Information can be extracted from the Internet or exchanged via the World Wide Web (www) by electronic mail, newsgroups and file transfer protocol (ftp). The World Wide Web is a system for providing access to a network of interlinked documents and information services across the Internet. Documents can be stored on the Web as text, images, sound or video. The language that the Web clients and servers use to communicate with each other is called 'hypertext transfer protocol' (http).

To use the World Wide Web you need software called a *browser* (or *client*) to view www documents, such as Navigator or Microsoft Internet Explorer. The latter is included with Windows, and the latest versions of both can be freely downloaded from the Web. If you want to read more about what informatics can do for you, read *The Clinician's Guide to Surviving IT*.[18]

There is now a large number of Internet Service Providers (ISPs), with the early ISPs such as AOL and CompuServe having been joined by others like BTInternet and TescoNet. The wide availability of broadband access has made using the Internet much more efficient and is rapidly superseding 'dial up'.

Medline

Medline is produced by the National Library of Medicine in the United States and is freely available to all (without a password) via the PubMed website: www.ncbi.nlm.nih.gov/entrez/query.fcgi?DB=pubmed

Other ways of searching Medline on the Web include the Dialog interface for all NHS staff * (ask your health library for a password or use the Athens self-registration function), or the Ebsco interface for university students or staff.

Medline contains over 12 million citations dating from 1950 to the present, from more than 4600 biomedical journals published in the United States and 70 other countries. Author abstracts are available for about 80% of the entries. It covers the whole field of medicine, dentistry, veterinary medicine, medical psychology, nursing, the healthcare system, and the pre-clinical sciences. Coverage is worldwide, but most records are from English-language sources or have English abstracts.

Cochrane Library

The Cochrane Library (www.library.nhs.uk) is considered to be the single best source of reliable evidence about the effects of healthcare.[19] The Cochrane Library includes:

- The Cochrane Database of Systematic Reviews (CDSR). These are structured, systematic reviews of controlled trials. Evidence is included or

* http://nhs.dialog.com/

excluded according to explicit quality criteria. A meta-analysis is under-taken by combining data from different studies to increase the *power* of the findings.
- The Database of Abstracts of Reviews of Effects (DARE). This is a database of research reviews of the effectiveness of healthcare interventions and the management and organisation of health services. The reviews are critically appraised by reviewers at the NHS Centre for Reviews and Dissemination at the University of York.
- The Cochrane Central Register of Controlled Trials (CENTRAL). This bib-liography of controlled trials has been compiled by both database and hand searches through the world's literature. The Register includes reports from conference proceedings.

This original core of the Cochrane Library has now been supplemented by the addition of: the NHS Economic Evaluation Database (NHSEED), Health Tech-nology Assessment Database (HTA) and Cochrane Methodology Register (CMR). The Cochrane Library was freely available to all via the National Library for Health (NLH) at: www.library.nhs.uk, but following the adoption of a new interface hosted by the publishers Wiley, access is currently restricted to the Database of Systematic Reviews only. Negotiations to restore full access are currently underway.

EMBASE

The Excerpta Medica database (EMBASE) is the largest competitor to Medline, but has a European bias in contrast to its rival's US bias. It contains over 7.5 million documents from 1974 to the present, indexed from over 4000 journals, and over 80% of entries have author abstracts. The overlap of coverage with Medline is around 40%, so a search on EMBASE will often recover papers not found on Medline. EMBASE has a similar subject coverage to Medline, but is stronger on pharmacology and therapeutics. Unlike Medline, which enjoys state subsidisation, EMBASE is produced commercially by the Dutch company Elsevier, and has consequently been too expensive in the past for all but the biggest of libraries to provide. However, EMBASE is now available as part of the NHSCore Content via Ovid (see your health library for a password).

CINAHL

The Cumulative Index to Nursing and Allied Health Literature (CINAHL) database, compiled by CINAHL Information Systems in the USA, is a compre-hensive database of more than 1200 English language journals from 1982 to the present. Some foreign language material has been included since 1994. CINAHL covers all aspects of nursing and allied health disciplines, such as health education, occupational therapy, physical therapy, emergency services, and social services and healthcare. Selected journals are also indexed in the areas of consumer health, biomedicine and health sciences librarianship. The database also provides access to healthcare books, nursing dissertations, selected conference proceedings, standards of professional practice, educational software and audio-visual materials in nursing. CINAHL has more than 7000 records with full text and 1200 records with images. Approximately 70% of CINAHL headings also appear in Medline. CINAHL supplements these headings with 4000+ terms designed specifically for nursing and allied health disciplines. For more information, see the following website: www.cinahl.com

Several studies have compared Medline and CINAHL. These revealed that while Medline assigns more index terms to each article, CINAHL uses index terms that are more focused on nursing and therapy topics.[20] Another study revealed that CINAHL was preferred by nursing students as it gave a higher number of relevant articles, while a further study found that both databases were relevant for allied health professionals (AHPs).[21,22] The authors concluded that, in order to ensure a comprehensive search, both Medline and CINAHL should be used. CINAHL is available via Ovid (see your health library for a password).

Subject-specific bibliographic databases[23,24]

Over 2 000 000 articles are published each year in over 20 000 medical and related journals. Thus, although electronic databases provide access to references from a large number of journals, no database provides access to all journals. So, if you search only one or two databases, you might miss a relevant article. In addition to searching the main databases, it is also worthwhile searching any specialist databases relevant to your area of interest. Some of these databases are outlined in alphabetical order below.

- **AgeLine** covers ageing, middle age and the elderly, and includes research on psychology, public policy, healthcare, business, gerontology and consumer issues. The information has a US bias but it is possible to limit to a particular target audience, e.g. patients or professionals. AgeLine is freely available at: http://research.aarp.org/ageline
- The databases formerly known as **AIDSDRUGS**, **AIDSTRIALS** and **AIDSLINE** are now searchable as a subset of PubMed via the NLM gateway at: http://gateway.nlm.nih.gov
- **AMED** (Allied and Alternative Medicine), available as part of the NHSCore Content via Ovid (see your health library for a password), searches across

the spectrum of complementary and alternative medicine. It covers articles from 400 journals, many of which are not indexed elsewhere, from 1985 to the present.

- **ASSIA plus** (Applied Social Sciences Index and Abstracts) covers all major social sciences and related media, including sociology, social policy, psychology and relevant aspects of anthropology, economics, medicine, law and politics. It features over 312 000 records from over 650 English language journals, covering 16 countries, including 25 of the 30 most cited sources. It covers the period since 1987 and is updated monthly. It is available (on subscription only) from Cambridge Scientific Abstracts Internet Database Service. See www.csa.com/factsheets/assia-set-c.php for more details.

- **CANCERLIT** – the database formerly known as CANCERLIT is now available as a subset of PubMed at www.cancer.gov/search/cancer_literature

- **Clinical Evidence** is a compendium of the best available evidence on the effects of common clinical interventions and is freely available to all via the National Library for Health (NLH) at: www.clinicalevidence.com/ceweb/conditions/index.jsp

- **EDINA BIOSIS** covers more than 6500 journals from more than 90 countries from 1985 to the present. It covers biological sciences and related subjects, including public health. It is updated every week and over 500 000 articles are added annually. EDINA offers the UK tertiary education and research community networked access to a library of data, information and research resources. All EDINA services were available free of charge to members of UK tertiary education institutions for academic use. Institutional subscription and personal registration is required. Go to the ISI Web of Knowledge Service for UK Education at: http://wos.mimas.ac.uk/

- The major online database for midwives is Maternity and Infant Care from MIDIRS (Midwives Information and Resource Service). This is available only from OVID (not Dialog) and access is dependent on whether your particular institution's ATHENS password allows it. The database contains over 120 000 references and unlike Medline includes material from non-journal sources such as books and the 'grey literature' (i.e. that which is not conventionally published). Coverage is from 1971 to date. More information is provided by the OVID datasheet at www.ovid.com/site/catalog/DataBase/2694.jsp

  Individuals (rather than institutions) can gain access by subscribing to the MIDIRS On Line Service (details at www.midirs.org/midirs/midweb1.nsf/services?openform)

- **PsycINFO**® includes worldwide literature from 1887 to the present in the field of psychology and psychological aspects of related disciplines, including medicine, psychiatry, nursing, sociology, education, pharmacology, physiology, linguistics, anthropology, business and law. PsycINFO is updated monthly and covers 1 300 journals in 25 languages – over 45 000 references are added annually. PsycINFO is available as part of the NHS Core Content via Ovid (see your health library for a password).

- **SUMSearch** is a unique method for searching the Internet for EBM information. It queries a variety of databases including Medline, the National Guideline Clearinghouse from the Agency for Health Care Policy and Research (AHCPR) and DARE. SUMSearch automatically corrects common abbreviations and common terms that are hard to search for on common databases. For example, it converts *DVT* to *deep vein thrombosis* and *heart failure* to *heart failure or ventricular failure* – small changes that greatly affect Medline search results. It is freely available at: http://sumsearch.uthscsa.edu

Other information on the Internet[23,24]

- **Bath Information and Data Service (BIDS)**[18] at www.bids.ac.uk is a database designed to be used by non-expert searchers and includes several medically orientated databases such as EMBASE, Citation Indexes and Inside Information, with a wide variety of medically related reference material. BIDS is at present only available to staff and students in the higher education community. As well as providing database access free at the point of delivery, a large number of full-text electronic journals, with links to database search results in many cases, are also available.
- **Health on the Net** at www.hon.ch The Health on the Net Foundation, a Swiss non-governmental organisation, has developed a code of conduct (HON code) for medical and health websites. This states that medical information should either be given by medically trained and qualified professionals or, if this is not possible, it should be indicated clearly that the information is given by non-medically qualified people. Websites complying with this code bear the Health on the Net logo. But the presence of a logo is not a guarantee of the quality of the information. A meta-search engine (one that searches many databases simultaneously) called MedHunt is supplied on the homepage.
- **Medical Matrix** at www.medmatrix.org This database is available only on subscription, lists over 6000 quality-assessed medical websites and links to over 1.5 million documents.
- The **National Research Register** (NRR) is a register of ongoing or recently completed research and development projects funded by, or of interest to, the NHS. It also contains details of reviews in progress collected by the NHS Centre for Reviews and Dissemination (CRD). The current

release (Issue 2 of 2006) contains information on 151 120 research projects, as well as entries from the Medical Research Council's Clinical Trials Directory. The NRR is assembled and published by Update Software Ltd on behalf of the Department of Health in the United Kingdom. The complete NRR database is free on the Internet at www.nrr.nhs.uk/search.htm
- **ReFeR**, the Department of Health Research Findings Register, helps to fill the gap between research completion and publication by providing details of the findings of many projects listed in the National Research Register. It is freely available via the NLH at: www.refer.nhs.uk/
- **PubMed** is the National Library of Medicine's search service that was developed in conjunction with publishers of biomedical literature as a search tool for accessing literature citations and linking to full-text journals at websites of participating publishers. It provides access to over 12 000 000 citations in Medline, PreMedline (updated daily, providing basic citation information and abstracts before the citation is indexed and added to Medline), NLM Gateway and other related databases, with links to participating online journals and textbooks. The NLM Gateway also gives access to OldMedline, which indexes journal articles from 1950 to 1965. Although searching PubMed is free, user registration, a subscription fee, or fee at the point of use may be required to access the full text of articles in some journals. It is available at www.ncbi.nlm.nih.gov/entrez/query.fcgi?DB=pubmed
- The **TRIP+** database is a one-stop search engine for evidence-based material on the Internet. Your higher education institution may have Athens access. www.tripdatabase.com

Website for learning evidence-based healthcare skills[25]

The Centre for Evidence-Based Medicine at Oxford includes a useful 'toolbox' and also downloads of free materials on its website at www.cebm.net/

Useful software

Mentor Plus[26] is an electronic medical knowledge clinical support system originally developed by Oxford University Press with EMIS (Egton Medical Information Systems Ltd). It has information about more than 2000 diseases cross-referenced with about 26 000 commonly used medical terms. The programme comes up with a differential diagnosis for a set of symptoms, signs and test results, suggesting appropriate management plans which are a mix of evidence-based medicine and best practice. EMIS is now offering an updated version, 'Web Mentor Libary' as a subscription service costing at present £74 plus VAT per annum.

Electronic journals

The situation regarding access to the full text of online journals is complicated and ever-changing. Ask your healthcare librarian for details. Some of the websites show the full contents of the journal, others do not carry the full text of all original articles.

*   *British Medical Journal* www.bmj.com (is now freely available for the current issue only, although your institution may have Athens access to full text).

As part of the NHS Core Content package, Proquest and some other agents provide access to over 1200 full-text journals. Ask your health library for an Athens password to use this service.

Higher education users will have access to a different package of electronic journals, usually needing an Athens password. Your university or college library can provide details.

'The greatest obstacle to discovering the truth is being convinced that you already know it.'

Stage 1

Asking the right question[27]

Although you may be burning to ask your question, when you actually try to set it down on paper, you may find that the exercise is more difficult than you think.

Questions have to be phrased in a very specific way to obtain meaningful responses in any context. This applies to asking other people what they think about a topic as much as for searching the literature for the best evidence.

The best clinical questions relate to queries arising from your own patients during the course of your work rather than being hypothetical questions. Relevant work-based questions should motivate you to seek the evidence and make change(s). Before you go to a lot of trouble to find answers or solutions to your questions, ask around at work and find out if anyone else is concerned about the same question or problem, already has the answer(s), or knows where to find them.

The question should be:

- simple
- specific
- realistic
- important
- capable of being answered
- agreed and owned by those who will be involved in any changes resulting
- implementable
- about a topic where change will be possible.

Think about how to construct your clinical question by considering:

- what the question is about. For example, is the question about an individual or group of patients? What are the patient characteristics you are interested in, such as age or gender? Is it a clinical dilemma or a resource problem?
- the setting. For example, is it specific to primary, secondary or community care, rural or urban locations?
- the type of intervention and whether it is being compared with current practice or another intervention. For example, are you interested in different treatments, causes, prognostic factors or risks, compared with current practice or no treatment?

- the outcome(s) of the clinical topic. For example, is an acceptable outcome to your question reduced numbers of cases of diseases, reduced patients' suffering, or increased quality of life?

You should focus and phrase your question to include whatever it is that you want to know about effects, efficiency, diagnosis or prognosis. You may decide to have a main question with several subsidiary questions.

Questions about cost-effectiveness

Cost-effectiveness is not synonymous with 'cheap'. A cost-effective intervention is one which gives a better or equivalent benefit from the intervention in question for lower or equivalent cost, or where the relative improvement in outcome is higher than the relative difference in cost. In other words, being cost-effective means having the best outcomes for the least input. Using the term 'cost-effective' implies that you have considered potential alternatives.

An intervention must first be considered *clinically* effective to warrant investigation into its potential to be *cost*-effective. Evidence-based practice must incorporate clinical judgement. You have to interpret the evidence when it comes to applying it to individual patients, whether it be evidence about clinical effectiveness or cost-effectiveness.

If you want to ask a question about cost-effectiveness you should be sure to have confirmed clinical effectiveness first, and have gone on to ask a question about cost-effectiveness as the second stage in seeking the evidence.

A 'benefit' is what is gained from meeting a chosen need and a 'cost' is the benefit that would have been obtained from using the same resources in an alternative way. Opportunity costs are the costs of the benefits foregone in deploying resources in the chosen way. They are the value of the benefits given up in the next best use of those resources.[28]

A new or alternative treatment or intervention should be compared directly with the next best treatment or intervention.

An economic evaluation is a comparative analysis of two or more alternatives in terms of their costs and consequences.[28,29] There are four different types: cost-effectiveness, cost minimisation, cost–utility analysis and cost–benefit analysis. Cost-effectiveness analysis is used to compare the effectiveness of two interventions with the same treatment objectives. Cost minimisation compares the costs of alternative treatments which have identical health outcomes. Cost–utility analysis enables the effects of alternative interventions to be measured against a combination of life expectancy and quality of life, a common outcome measure being 'quality-adjusted life-years' (QALYs). A cost–benefit analysis compares the incremental costs and benefits of a programme.

Efficiency is sometimes confused with effectiveness. Being efficient means having obtained the most quality from the least expenditure, or the required level of quality for the least expenditure. To measure efficiency you need to make a judgement about the level of quality of the 'purchase' and be able to relate it to 'price'. 'Price' alone does not measure efficiency. Quality is the indicator used in combination with price to assess whether something is more efficient.

So, cost-effectiveness is a measure of efficiency and suggests that costs have been related to effectiveness.

> 'I have finally made up my mind but the decision was by no means unanimous.'

Framing questions: some examples

Now try these two examples of clinical situations and frame a specific question for each with which you might search the literature for evidence to answer the questions.

Jot down notes under each heading and write the final question at the bottom of the page ready to do a trial literature search using the Medline database. Refine and limit the question to one which would seem to be relevant for midwives delivering maternity services. Your question should be shaped by thinking out exactly why you are asking it and how you might apply the evidence in practice once you have obtained it.

Set a question to address problem 1

An antenatal clinic is taking stock of the preventive work it does and is reviewing whether to continue the range of work that different health professionals provide. The community midwives and other staff are wondering what the impact is of the range of health education about smoking that they offer their patients.

1 What is the question about – an individual patient, a group of people, a particular population, patient characteristics, a clinical dilemma, a resource problem?
2 What is the setting or context of the clinical topic/situation?
3 Is there an intervention and, if so, with what is it being compared?
4 What is/are the outcome(s) of the clinical topic?
5 What is the specific question you will ask?

6   Choose up to four key words in priority order that you think best represent the important components of your question and that will restrict it as far as possible to your field of enquiry.

Some example details follow.

Example details of question posed to address problem 1

Defining the question

The refined question should narrow down the limits of the enquiry by specifying as many of the following details as apply:

- What is the question about – the whole or a section of the practice population? What is meant by health education? Which staff are involved with the health education intervention? What is meant by 'smoking', etc?
- What is the setting or context of the enquiry? The focus of your interest might be antenatal care, postnatal care or the impact of smoking on the neonate.
- Is there an intervention and, if so, with what is it being compared? What types of health education is the questioner interested in? Is there an alternative model to which health education is being compared?
- What is/are the outcome(s) of the health education intervention and what is meant by 'impact', e.g. changes in attitudes, quantity of cigarettes smoked, reduction in detriment to health?
- The specific question will have narrowed down the problem to one in which the midwives are interested. For instance, if midwives were reviewing whether to continue the pre-conception clinic, besides looking at attendance figures, patient preferences, and opportunity costs for staff, the midwives might want to know 'What is the evidence for the effectiveness of face-to-face education about the risks of cigarette smoking in midwife-run clinics?' A more general question might be 'What is the evidence for the effectiveness of a health professional advising a smoker to stop smoking?'
- Key words might be health education, smoking, maternity, etc., depending on your question. You might have other key words.

If you try this exercise with other midwives you may find that you all compose entirely different questions as you have different foci of interests. Some may find that their question does not contain the key words they selected after finalising their question, as they had not refined their ideas sufficiently. If they were to go on to search on their chosen key words on Medline that would miss the point of their various questions.

Set a question to address problem 2

A pregnant woman asks her midwife if she should try acupuncture for her early morning sickness and if it will reduce her constant nausea.

Have a go at completing parts of the question for problem 2.

1 What is the question about – an individual patient, a group of people, a particular population, patient characteristics, a clinical dilemma, a resource problem?
2 What is the setting or context of the clinical topic/situation?
3 Is there an intervention and, if so, with what is it being compared?
4 What is/are the outcome(s) of the clinical topic?
5 What is the specific question you will ask?
6 Choose up to four key words in priority order that you think best represent the important components of your question and that will restrict them as far as possible to your field of enquiry.

Some example details follow.

Example details of question posed to address problem 2

Defining the question

A refined question will narrow down the limits of the enquiry by specifying as many of the following details as apply:

- What is the question about – the woman or all pregnant women suffering from morning sickness, e.g. nausea, vomiting, or both? What is meant by morning sickness? What is meant by acupuncture?
- What is the setting or context of the enquiry? The focus of your interest might be antenatal clinics, the community or primary care.
- If there is an intervention, with what is it being compared – the method of acupuncture, or any other type of intervention for morning sickness?
- What is/are the outcome(s) of the intervention and what is meant by reduce – changes in nausea symptoms, reduction in frequency of vomiting?
- The specific question should narrow down the problem to one in which the woman and midwife are interested. So you might ask 'what is the evidence for the effectiveness of acupuncture point stimulation in controlling nausea and vomiting associated with morning sickness?'
- Key words might be acupuncture, nausea, morning sickness, pregnancy. You might have other key words.

Examples of questions you might pose as a midwife

These are not given as examples that show particularly good or bad question formats; they are included here to show the range and variety of questions that individual midwives might develop as part of their work. We include examples of evidence they might find, then interpret and decide whether or not to put that evidence into practice.

Q: What are the effects of preventive interventions in women at high risk of pre-eclampsia?
The evidence: 'Anti-platelet drugs (mainly aspirin) reduce the risk of pre-eclampsia ... calcium supplementation reduces the relative risk of pre-eclampsia by about a third.' There is 'insufficient evidence on the effects of fish oil, or of evening primrose oil plus fish oil or calcium on the risk of pre-eclampsia and preterm birth.'[30]

Q: What are the effects of interventions in women who develop hypertension in pregnancy?
The evidence: There is 'limited evidence from which it is not possible to demonstrate benefit for hospital admission, bed rest or day care compared with outpatient care.' ... It is unclear whether women with mild to moderate hypertension during pregnancy derive benefit from antihypertensive drugs.' ... 'For women with severe hypertension during pregnancy, antihypertensive drugs will lower blood pressure.' There is 'promising evidence that magnesium sulphate may reduce the risk of developing eclampsia, but other possible benefits and harms are unclear.'[30]

Q: What is the best choice of anticonvulsant for women with eclampsia?
The evidence: '... magnesium sulphate reduced the risk of further fits in women with eclampsia compared with phenytoin, diazepam, or lytic cocktail.'[30]

Q: What are the effects of preventive interventions in women at high risk of preterm delivery?
The evidence: 'Antibiotic treatment of bacterial vaginosis during pregnancy decreases the incidence of preterm delivery, especially in women who have had a previous preterm delivery.' There is no evidence that 'enhanced antenatal care reduces the risk of preterm delivery.' In women 'presumed to have cervical incompetence, cervical cerclage is associated with a significant reduction in preterm births (less than 33 weeks gestation).'[30]

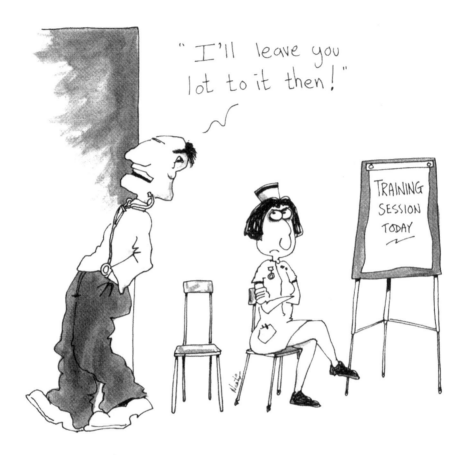

Clinical effectiveness is done best by involving the whole team.

Stage 2

Undertaking a literature search

The search strategy: think, search and appraise

A search for the best evidence follows the sequence of 'think, search and appraise'. This search strategy comprises:

- thinking about and defining a good specific question in consultation with all the staff who are involved in the question and affected by possible change(s)
- searching for and finding the best level of evidence by looking critically at the relevant publications obtained
- appraising and interpreting the evidence as applied to your question in relation to your situation.

Clinical effectiveness encompasses the whole cycle:

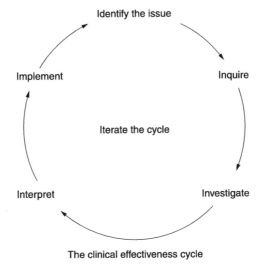

The clinical effectiveness cycle

Figure 1:   The clinical effectiveness cycle.

It is tempting for midwives who are pushed for time and hot on the scent of evidence with which to answer a question to jump straight from an idea to carrying out a search, instead of working through the steps with the necessary rigour. Cutting corners wastes time in the long run if you ask the wrong question, answer a different question to the one you intended, or become distracted by lots of interesting but irrelevant literature.

How long you spend and to what lengths you go with a search will depend on its purpose. If you were commissioned to undertake a major systematic review, you would spend many months searching every relevant database, hand searching through papers and journals, hunting up conference proceedings, trying personal contacts, translating non-English language papers, and generally leaving no stone unturned in the pursuit of published and unpublished studies. But as you are probably a busy clinician who just wants to find the best evidence for answering a question in practice, you should strictly limit your search as your resources are limited. You will probably be better off spending your precious time doing several searches for different topics than doing one exhaustive search on a single subject. So stop your search if you find a relevant systematic review of multiple, well-designed, randomised controlled trials in the Systematic Reviews section of the Cochrane Library. If there is no such systematic review move on to look for a review in the Database of Abstracts of Reviews of Effects (DARE). If no luck there try Medline, or EMBASE, or other specialist databases until you obtain the best possible level of evidence that you can find.

If you have not undertaken a search of the literature before, you would be well advised to book an individual session with your local healthcare librarian and to undertake a search in your health library if this is possible. You should be able to teach yourself from guidebooks, these notes, and trial and error, but a healthcare librarian is the person with the know-how about the best thesaurus terms and phrases to try with your search. You as a health professional will know about the validity, context and relevance of search words and phrases as applied to your question. Together, you as a clinician or other professional and the healthcare librarian make a strong search team.

Undertake a search

Before you start, *write down* the key words you want to use, putting them in order of importance. How many key words you enter at the first stage depends on how wide you expect your field of enquiry to be. If you key in *asthma*, you would expect to identify thousands more references to published papers than if you keyed in the name of a rare condition. So if you are searching within a broad topic area such as *asthma* you should prepare more potential words to narrow the field of your search for the few most relevant papers that will supply evidence to answer your original question. Refine your question prior to your search so that it is very focused and make sure that the key words are the most pertinent you can manage. Then you will spend less time on your search and have more chance of finding the most appropriate published evidence. So if you want to know more in the subject area of *asthma*, build your question carefully. Aim specifically at the purpose of the question and include the setting, the population under question, the intervention, the outcome and any other important details.

Using the Cochrane Library

Enter your most important key words first. Look at the different levels of evidence from the systematic reviews on the Cochrane Database of Systematic Reviews (CDSR) to controlled trials on the Cochrane Central Register of Controlled Trials (CENTRAL) to the abstracts on the Database of Abstracts of Reviews of Effects (DARE). The hierarchy of evidence is explained further in the next section. You may find that you have access only to CDSR.

It is likely that you will obtain only a small number of relevant-sounding systematic reviews, because this part of the Cochrane Library contains a relatively small number of specially written comprehensive reviews, rather than references to individual journal articles, as is the case in, for example, Medline. It is more likely that you will not find a relevant systematic review, but will identify many references to controlled trials. You should then modify your search by entering the first words again plus an extra key word that was your next choice in order of priority. If this does not refine your search enough, repeat the exercise, adding a fourth key word. When you have narrowed your search sufficiently, obtain copies of the original articles as appropriate so that you can critically appraise them yourself.

Do not assume that the contents of any paper published in a journal are valid, reliable or accurate, however reputable the journal. Mistakes may have been overlooked, studies reported might not be relevant to your own situation, or the results may not be generalisable to your question.

If your search on the Cochrane Library was unsuccessful, try another database with a larger number of individual references, such as Medline.

Using the Medline database

Because Medline contains an enormous number of references you will have to develop a very strict search strategy to narrow down your focus of enquiry. To search on Medline, a good starting point is to use the terms in its thesaurus, the Medical Subject Heading list (MeSH). There are over 17 500 MeSH terms arranged as a tree structure with broad subject areas branching off and subdividing into narrower subject terms. If you use a word which is not a MeSH heading,

Medline suggests an alternative. For instance if you type 'primary care', Medline suggests 'primary health care'. If you type 'cigarettes', 'smoking' is suggested.

Medline may be searched either by key word(s) in the title or abstract, or by selected headings from the MeSH list.

Entering one key word will often yield thousands of references, but a more selective search is possible by combining key words using 'and' and 'or' (these are called Boolean operators). To narrow the search further you can restrict the date range, the language the paper is written in, to 'Priority Journals' (an abridged list), or to 'human' as opposed to 'animal' research.

In a healthcare library, all you will need to do to access Medline or the Cochrane Library is to ask a member of staff. Your Athens password will also allow you to use your home (or any Internet-enabled) computer to search the databases.

Try an easy-to-follow practical detail of undertaking a Medline search,[31] which you could consult if you are unfamiliar with Medline searching and want to read more about the process before having a go for yourself.

Hints for the use of Medline are:

*   click on a **Subject Heading** to view its position in the hierarchical 'Tree'
*   select the **Explode** box to retrieve references indexed under your selected MeSH heading plus all the more specific terms stemming from it
*   select the **Focus** box to limit your search to those documents in which your MeSH heading is considered to be the main point of the article.

You will learn most by having a go. You really cannot do anything wrong that you are not able to put right by retracing your steps.

The hierarchy of evidence

The table below shows one of the common ways of grading the evidence ranging from level I, which is the most robust evidence, to level V, based on the opinions of experts in the field.[27] There may not be any strong evidence in the literature for answering the question(s) you are posing.

Type	Evidence
I	Strong evidence from at least one systematic review of multiple, well-designed, randomised controlled trials
II	Strong evidence from at least one properly designed, randomised controlled trial of appropriate size
III	Evidence from well-designed trials without randomisation, single group pre–post, cohort, time series or matched case–control studies
IV	Evidence from well-designed non-experimental studies from more than one centre or research group
V	Opinions of respected authorities, based on clinical evidence, descriptive studies or reports of expert committees

The most valid types of research for extracting evidence about clinical effectiveness are randomised controlled trials, followed by controlled trials not using randomisation, then uncontrolled trials and, less reliably, observational studies. A systematic review of several randomised controlled trials of all known studies is better than a review of some studies, which in turn is better than a case study. You should start to search for the best evidence and, if you do not find it, work down the hierarchy.

If there is no reliable evidence to be found after searching the Cochrane Library, Medline and other relevant databases, you should then move on to look for any expert consensus agreements by multidisciplinary groups.

Be realistic – try to find one or a few key reviews rather than get bogged down in a plethora of papers. Clinical effectiveness is a tool for keeping up to date, enhancing your clinical practice, and retaining your professional interest – spending too much time pursuing it may be counterproductive.

> 'Most of my problems either have no answer or else the answer is worse than the problem.'

Examples

Example of literature search using problem 1 described previously

Question: What is the evidence for the effectiveness of a midwife advising a pregnant woman to stop smoking?

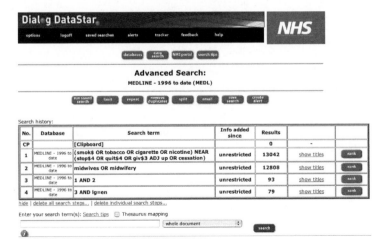

The key to an effective search is to anticipate the likely words used in the title, abstract, or controlled vocabulary (MeSH in the case of Medline) headings of any relevant papers.

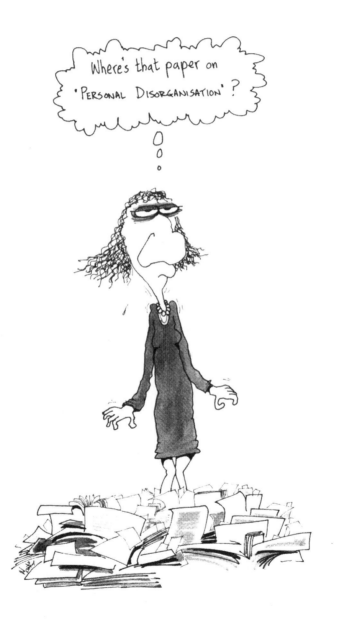

Use IT to ask a question and search for the evidence systematically.

Using MeSH headings alone will miss the most recent material, which appears on the database before it is fully indexed (i.e. before MeSH headings have been assigned).

NB. Much better results will be obtained by combining individual words than by attempting to ask a 'natural language' question such as "How effective is the advice of a midwife in stopping pregnant women smoking?" Doing this will simply 'confuse' the search engine.

The first line of the search strategy uses two important techniques to improve the sensitivity (i.e. how many potentially useful papers are identified) of the search. The first is called 'truncation'. For example, 'smok$' finds the words 'smoke(s)', 'smoked' or 'smoking' without having to enter the words individually. The dollar sign ($) after the stem of the word means 'find this stem, plus any numbers of letters following it'.

In the same way, 'stop$4' ('stop$' returns an error message saying: "too many terms in truncation") finds 'stop(s)', 'stopped', or 'stopping' and 'quit$' finds 'quit(s)' or 'quitting'.

The second technique is the use of the operator 'NEAR'. This finds words occurring within five words of each other and in any order. In the example given, the use of 'NEAR' means that the phrase 'stopping smoking' would be found, as would 'smoking cessation', 'giving up smoking' or 'quitting cigarettes'.

The Dialog search engine automatically allows for both the singular and plural of any word to be searched for, so entering 'midwives' on the second line of the search also finds 'midwife'.

The Cochrane Library can be searched using exactly the same search words, but the truncation sign changes from a dollar sign ($) to an asterisk (*). Use the 'Advanced Search' option.

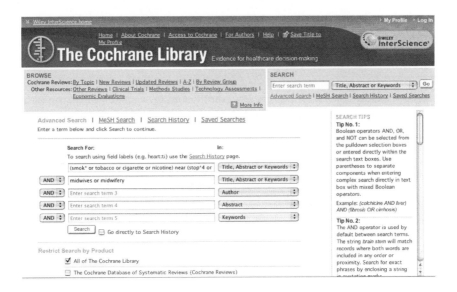

Example of literature search using problem 2 described previously

Question: What are the effects of interventions to improve outcome after preterm rupture of the membranes?

Any paper relevant to this question will almost certainly include the words 'premature' or 'preterm' in the title or abstract. Sometimes 'preterm' is hyphenated and appears as 'pre-term'. The Dialog search engine uses the hyphen to indicate a multi-word thesaurus (MeSH) heading, so you should not use it yourself.

Simply leaving a space where the hyphen would be means that Dialog treats 'pre term' as a phrase (words appearing adjacent to each other) and automatically introduces 'ADJ' to indicate this. As you saw in the first example, using truncation and the 'NEAR' operator means that the phrases 'premature rupture' and 'ruptured prematurely' will both be found.

The 'NEAR' operator is used again in the second line of the search strategy ('membranes'), ensuring that the word order of any phrases searched for becomes unimportant.

Adding the word 'outcome' (the relevant MeSH heading is 'TREATMENT OUTCOME', so this is automatically included in the search results) refines the results, but still leaves you with too many to look through easily.

As you are trying to find the best possible evidence, a simple but effective way of doing this is to search for 'random$ or systematic or metaanalysis or meta analysis' and combine this with your results. This will identify any randomised controlled trials, systematic reviews, or meta-analyses.

Once again, the same strategy can be used for searching the Cochrane Library, remembering only to substitute the asterisk for the dollar sign when using truncation.

Advanced Search:
MEDLINE - 1996 to date (MEDL)

[run saved search] [limit] [repeat] [remove duplicates] [split] [email] [save search] [create alert]

Search history:

No.	Database	Search term	Info added since	Results		
CP		[Clipboard]		0	-	
1	MEDLINE - 1996 to date	(premature OR preterm OR pre ADJ term) NEAR rupture$	unrestricted	2376	show titles	rank
2	MEDLINE - 1996 to date	membranes	unrestricted	390105	show titles	rank
3	MEDLINE - 1996 to date	1 NEAR 2	unrestricted	2318	show titles	rank
4	MEDLINE - 1996 to date	outcome	unrestricted	572920	show titles	rank
5	MEDLINE - 1996 to date	3 AND 4	unrestricted	1016	show titles	rank
6	MEDLINE - 1996 to date	random$ OR systematic OR metaanalysis OR meta ADJ analysis	unrestricted	408967	show titles	rank
7	MEDLINE - 1996 to date	5 AND 6	unrestricted	192	show titles	rank
8	MEDLINE - 1996 to date	7 AND lg=en	unrestricted	180	show titles	rank

hide | delete all search steps... | delete individual search steps...

Enter your search term(s): Search tips ☐ Thesaurus mapping

[   ]   [whole document   ÷]   [search]

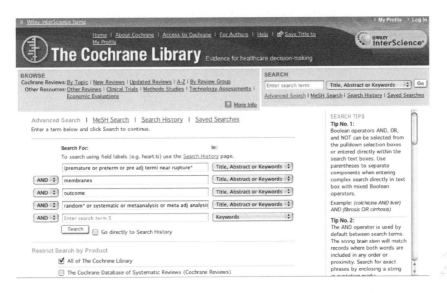

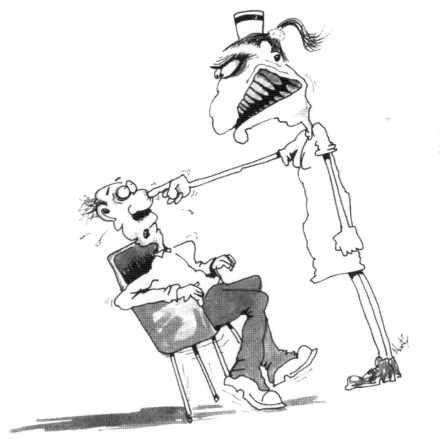

Information is power!

Searching by yourself

Now you do it – work through an example by yourself.

1 Take any one (or both) of two problems which interests you most – whether health education on smoking is worth doing, or whether a breech presenting at term should be managed by external cephalic version. Adapt the problem(s) to your own circumstances. The idea of this exercise is that you will run a search on a question (or questions) similar to the ones already described so that you can follow the procedures laid out in this book for guidance, but adapted to your own situation so that it is more relevant to you. Conducting your own version of the search will give you more confidence that you can do a literature search yourself. Write in your own words what your perspective of the problem is:

2 Frame the words of your question to address that problem - the words you use in the question should vary from any presented in this book, as the angle of the problem and the focus of the question should relate to your own circumstances. Write in your own words what the question is:

3 Choose up to five key words and put them in order of priority:

4 Undertake a search for the evidence to answer that problem. If possible go to your healthcare library and book time with a healthcare librarian and the computerised search facilities there. Use the Cochrane database first and then Medline.

Cochrane search

• Write down how you will use your key words to search the Cochrane Library. Which one, two or three words will you key in first? Then, which words will you add, and in what order, to narrow the focus of your search?

- How did the search go? How many 'hits' did you obtain from the Cochrane Library?
  - systematic reviews on the Cochrane Database of Systematic Reviews (CDSR):
    (i) number of reviews =
    (ii) number of protocols =
  - controlled trials on the Cochrane Central Register of Controlled Trials (CENTRAL) =
  - abstracts on the Database of Abstracts of Reviews of Effects (DARE) =

- Print off up to five references that seem relevant to your question, so that you can obtain the original papers if you should wish to. Print off the abstracts if you have the facilities to do so.

Medline search

- Write down how you will use your key words to search the Medline database. Which one, two or three words will you key in first? Then, which words will you add, and in what order, to narrow the focus of your search?

- Begin your search and key the words in, exploding, combining and modifying the search according to the order of key words you have just specified and the numbers of papers you obtain at each stage. Go back to the instructions about using Medline and work through the examples and helpful suggestions if you have difficulties doing your own search.

- How did the search go? Print off your search strategy, to provide a record of the separate stages of your search. If you cannot print the strategy, copy it down in the table below under the headings 'Set', 'Search' and 'Results'.

Set	Search	Results
1		

- When you get down to fewer than 100 or so articles, scroll through the abstracts on the screen and print off the details of the ones that seem most relevant.

- If you have still not obtained any relevant evidence, you have a choice of trying other databases, or following up references given in papers with content nearest to your field of enquiry, or contacting experts named as authors or investigators to find out if there is work in press or other publications you have missed, or any other pertinent information. If you already know of one relevant paper, try to find the Medline entry for it by searching under the author's name and combining it with a search for words in the title. When you have found it, examine the full record to see what MeSH terms the indexers have used. This may give you some ideas for other terms to search under.

You should not expect to find exactly the same results as in the examples given earlier, as not only will you have modified the problem, the linked question and the search strategy to fit your own circumstances, but the details of publications held on the Cochrane and Medline databases will have been added to over time.

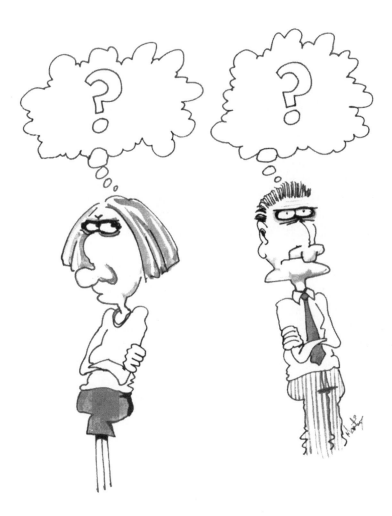

Choose a question that is important to you and your colleagues at work and where changes in practice will be possible.

Stage 3

Frame your own question and search for the evidence

Now that you have learned the theory behind doing a search and have seen how other midwives like you have framed their questions and searched for the evidence, you should be ready to shape your own question and find the best available evidence that exists.

1 Think about a problem at work which you consider would be an appropriate topic for this exercise. Consult others at work; do they think it is a problem too? Is it an important issue for them and do they think you would be spending your time wisely searching for evidence about best practice? Is there likely to be a change that you could make which would bring benefits to you, colleagues or patients, or result in a saving of resources? As this book is considering how to improve clinical effectiveness you should choose a clinical topic in this instance, but another time you might choose to search for evidence on a management issue. What is the problem you have chosen to investigate? Write it down here:

Who else did you consult before deciding on this problem?

What sort of changes at work do you have in mind that might be possible to put into action, depending on what evidence you find?

2 Frame the words of your question which addresses that problem. Build up the question as described previously, being as specific as possible, but not so specific that you narrow your field of enquiry and eliminate possible options that might be appropriate, such as novel types of intervention. Include the

purpose of the question, what it is about, the setting, the population and the outcome(s). Write in your own words what the question is:

Are there any subsidiary questions?

Have you discussed the question with anyone else? If so, with whom?

3   Choose up to five key words and put them in order of priority:

Are you satisfied that these key words reflect all the essential ingredients of your original problem and capture the essence of the question?

4   Undertake a search for the evidence to answer the question. If possible go to your health library and book time with a healthcare librarian who can help and advise you if necessary. Try the Cochrane Library first and then Medline.

Cochrane search

- Write down how you will use your key words to search the Cochrane Library. Which one, two or three words will you key in first? Then, which words will you add, and in what order, to narrow the focus of your search?

- How did the search go? How many 'hits' did you obtain from the Cochrane Library?
    - systematic reviews on the Cochrane Database of Systematic Reviews (CDSR):
      (i) number of reviews =
      (ii) number of protocols =
    - controlled trials on the Cochrane Central Register of Controlled Trials (CENTRAL) =
    - abstracts on the Database of Abstracts of Reviews of Effects (DARE) =

- Print off up to five sets of details of articles that seem relevant to your question. Print off the abstracts of these articles if you are able to do so. Obtain copies of the original papers.

Medline search

- Write down how you will use your key words to search the Medline database. Which one, two or three words will you key in first? Then, which words will you add, and in what order, to narrow the focus of your search?

- Begin your search and key the words in, exploding, combining and modifying the search according to the order of key words you have just specified and the numbers of papers you obtain at each stage.

- How did the search go? Print off the results of the search in the same way as the screenshots given as examples earlier listed the stages of the search, the modifications and the numbers of papers identified from the key words. If you cannot print the results off the screen, copy them down here under the headings 'Set', 'Search' and 'Results'.

Set	Search	Results
1		

- When you get down to fewer than 100 or so articles, scroll through the abstracts on the screen and print off the details of the ones that seem most relevant.

- If you have still not obtained any relevant evidence you have a choice of trying other databases, or following up references given in papers with content nearest to your field of enquiry, or contacting experts named as authors or investigators to find out if there is work in press or other publications you have missed, or any other pertinent information. If you already know of one relevant paper, try to find the Medline entry for it by searching under the author's name and combining it with a search for words in the title. When you have found it, examine the full record to see what MeSH terms the indexers have used. This may give you some ideas for other terms to search under.

Save your search strategy for re-running at a later date. Once a strategy has been saved, it can be edited and lines added, deleted or changed as your ideas develop.

Stage 4

Appraise the evidence

Now that you have extracted the publications that seem most relevant to your own question from your search, the next steps are to decide how much reliance you can put on their contents and how far you can extrapolate from those papers to your own circumstances. This will involve deciding whether the studies described in the papers were well conducted or flawed, whether the population and setting studied were similar enough to your own circumstances for the results to be generalisable to your population or setting, whether sufficient people or things were studied for the results to be representative of larger numbers, and how you will weigh one paper against another if they report conflicting results or conclusions.

Critical appraisal is the assessment of evidence by systematically reviewing its validity and results, and relevance to specific situations.

Critical appraisal:

- identifies the strengths and weaknesses of a research paper
- develops a better understanding of scientific principles and research methodology
- increases capability to understand to what extent published literature is applicable to other circumstances.

The meaning of different research methods and terms

Some common research terms are outlined below. A wider glossary of terms is available online at www.jr2.ox.ac.uk/Bandolier/glossary.html

Bias

Systematic deviation of the results from the true results due to the way(s) in which the study was carried out.

Confidence intervals

This describes the degree of confidence that can be placed on any statistical result. It describes the range of results from the subjects or things studied within which the investigator is 95% certain that the true population mean lies (the usual level of confidence chosen).

Confounder or confounding factor

A factor, other than the variables under study, which is not controlled for and which distorts the results causing a spurious association.

Controlled trial

As for a randomised controlled trial (see relevant entry) without the randomisation element.

A controlled trial detects associations between an intervention and an outcome but does not rule out the possibility that the association was caused by an unrecognised third factor linking both the intervention and the outcome.

Controls

The subjects in a (randomised) controlled trial who are (randomly) allocated to receive either placebo, no treatment or the standard treatment.

Cost-effectiveness analysis (CEA)

Compares the effectiveness of two interventions with the same treatment objectives. Competing interventions are compared in terms of costs per unit of consequence. Consequences may vary but are measured in monetary terms.

Cost–benefit analysis (CBA)

Compares the incremental costs and benefits of a programme. Measures both costs and benefits in monetary values and calculates net monetary gains or losses (presented as a cost–benefit ratio).

Cost-minimisation analysis (CMA)

Compares the costs of alternative treatments that have identical outcomes.

Cost–utility analysis (CUA)

Measures the effects of alternative interventions in terms of a combination of life expectancy and quality of life, using utility measures such as quality-adjusted life-years (QALYs), and may present relative costs per QALY.

Efficacy

The extent to which an intervention produces a beneficial result under ideal conditions. Preferably based on a randomised controlled trial (RCT).

Effectiveness

The extent to which an intervention does what it is intended to do for a defined population.

Hawthorne effect

The influence of knowledge of the study on behaviour. The effect of being in a study on the persons being studied.

Incidence

The numbers or proportion of new cases of a disease or condition occurring within a population over a given period of time.

Intention to treat analysis

This is a quantitative estimate of the benefit of a therapy in the population being studied derived from comparing control and treatment groups.

Numbers needed to treat (NNT) are being cited in published papers increasingly commonly. You need to know the characteristics of the population being studied, the disease and its severity, the treatment and its duration, the comparator and the outcomes.

Meta-analysis

This is a method of combining two or more studies to obtain information about larger numbers of subjects. Inclusion criteria should be clearly stated in the method to enable different studies to be considered together. It should appear reasonable to treat the sum of the different studies as one whole and that like is being combined with like.

Observational study

There are several types of study where the subjects are observed over time and the experiences are recorded or reported.

A cohort study is one where two similar groups of people who do not have the disease or condition under study are observed prospectively over a predetermined period to see the effects of one group being exposed to an already established suspected risk factor (such as cigarette smoking) and the other group not being so exposed.

A cross-sectional survey gathers information about subjects or things in a study population at one point in time or over a relatively short period.

Odds ratio (OR)

A measure of treatment effectiveness. The probability of an event happening as opposed to it not happening. An OR of 1 means that the effects of treatment are no different from no treatment. If the OR is greater than (or less than) 1, it means that the effects of treatment are more (or less) than those of the control group.

Placebo

An inert substance that is given to control subjects in trials.

Power

Sample sizes should be calculated before the study design is finalised to determine the numbers needed to be likely to detect a sufficient effect from the study intervention, so as to be sure that the effect did not occur by chance alone. The power calculation predicts the number that needs to be studied to detect an effect at least at the level of 95% significance. This is the level of certainty that is equal to or less than a one in 20 risk that the effect occurred by chance and was not due to an intervention or event being studied.

Prevalence

The proportion of 'cases' within a specified population at a given time.

Probability

Probabilities are often written as p values in published reports, where p stands for probability. It is a measure of how likely an outcome is. This lies between 0 (where an event will never happen) and 1.0 (where it will definitely occur).

The p value is a guide to the likelihood that the outcome measured occurred by chance or was due to the intervention or event that the study was designed to measure.

A significant p value is one where the likelihood is that the effect or outcome occurred as a result of the intervention or event being studied, and did not occur by chance. The most common convention is to decide arbitrarily on a one in 20 risk of being wrong about the direct causal relationship between the intervention or event and the outcome; that is, the risk that the outcome occurred by chance. This can be described as '$p = 0.05$', 'at the 5% significance level' or as a '5 in 100 probability' that the outcome occurred by chance. If written as '$p < 0.05$' there is less than a 5 in 100 risk of the outcome having happened by chance. Smaller p values give increased confidence in the test results; for example $p < 0.001$ indicates that the probability that the outcome occurred by chance is less than one in a thousand. The level of significance the investigators choose should depend on the importance of being right about the intervention/outcome relationship, and the numbers in the populations being studied.

Sometimes investigators get carried away, testing every bit of data in their study to see if they can dredge up some significant results. This is very bad practice because even a short questionnaire can yield hundreds of combinations of possibilities if each question has several alternative categories of answer, for example age might be subdivided into nine decades. If a signifi-cance test was applied to all the possible combinations of answers looking for potential links and 200 tests of significance were tried, for example, you would expect ten tests erroneously to indicate statistical significance where the outcome(s) had occurred by chance (that is, a 5 in 100 risk $\times$ 2 = 10). So the arbitrary $p < 0.05$ test of assumed significance is not cut-and-dried proof that an outcome is directly attributable to an intervention – it is just a good indicator of significance.

Publication bias

Results are more likely to be published if the results are positive rather than negative. Thus, it may appear that treatments have more positive results than is actually the case.

Randomised controlled trial (RCT)

Randomisation is necessary to minimise and, hopefully, eliminate selection bias. This is the type of study design which is most likely to give you a true result because only one section of the subjects or things in the trial are exposed to the intervention or factor being studied. The subjects or things are randomly allocated either to the group exposed to the intervention or to the control group, who are not intentionally exposed to that intervention. The experiences and outcomes of both groups are compared to see if they are significantly different according to statistical tests. Sometimes the design includes more than two comparative groups.

Using the randomised controlled trial method distributes unsuspected bio-logical variables equally between the two groups, as well as any other external factors of which you are unaware. Both the subject and control groups will be exposed to these unrecognised external influences (called confounding factors) and any differences in outcomes between the two groups should be attribu-table to the intervention being studied.

When the term 'randomised' is stated there should be some information in the method as to how this randomisation process was carried out to minimise any external influences from interfering with the random allocation of subjects or things to different arms of the study.

If a trial is 'double blind', neither the clinician/investigator giving the treatment or analysing the results, nor the person receiving it, should know whether they are in the treatment or the control group. In a 'single' blind study, either the clinician or the subject knows what treatment the subject is receiving.

Relative risk

Relative risk is calculated by taking the ratio between two measures of risk. If there is no difference between two groups the risk ratio is '1', as the risks in each group are the same. A risk ratio greater than '1' shows the outcome in the study group to be better than that for controls.

   The risk ratio is the proportion of the group at risk in one group divided by the proportion at risk in a second group. The risk ratio is a measure of relative risk.

Reliability

A reliable method is one which produces repeatable results.

Sensitivity of test

The true positive rate of a diagnostic test, that is, how often the test misses people with the disease.

Sensitivity analysis

Tests the robustness of the results of an economic analysis by varying the underlying assumptions around which there is uncertainty.

Specificity of test

The true negative rate of a diagnostic test, that is, how often the test indicates people as having the disease when they do not.

Statistically significant

By convention taken to be at the 5% level ($p < 0.05$). This means that the observed result would occur by chance in only one in 20 cases (*see* Probability).

Systematic review

Systematic reviews of randomised controlled trials provide the highest level of evidence of the effectiveness of treatments – preventative, therapeutic and rehabilitatory treatments (as described in the section on hierarchy of evidence, p 28).

Validity

A valid method is one which measures what it sets out to measure.

Reading a paper

Reading and evaluating a paper is mainly about applying common sense. Traditionally, critical appraisal of the literature has been made to seem like a difficult science for the elite, rather than a basic skill that any health professional can readily learn and apply to their own situation.

If you read the summary of a research study overleaf and answer the questions, you will soon discover for yourself some of the common flaws in published studies, sometimes even those in respected peer-reviewed journals where the mistakes were not noted by the researchers or publication team.

In general you should consider whether:

- the paper is relevant to your own practice
- the research question is well defined
- any definitions are unambiguous
- the aim(s) and/or objective(s) of the study are clearly stated
- the design and methodology are appropriate for the aim(s) of the study
- the measuring instruments seem to be reliable; that is, different observers at different points in time would arrive at the same outcome
- the measuring instruments seem to be valid; that is, the investigator is actually measuring that which she/he intends to measure
- the sampling method is clear
- the results relate to the aim(s) and objective(s) of the study
- the results seem to be robust and justifiable
- the results can be generalised to your own circumstances
- there are any biases in the method of the study
- there are biases in the results, such as non-reporting of drop-outs from the study
- the conclusion is valid
- you have any other concerns about the study.

Specifically you should look at:

- where the study was done and who are the authors
- the study design: how were the subjects and controls selected, were they randomised and if so how, what were the outcome measures, were the outcome measures clinically relevant, are the sample numbers appropriate?
- the results: are the numbers of drop-outs and non-respondents reported, are all subjects accounted for, is the statistical analysis explained, are the results clearly presented?
- the discussion and conclusions: does the report describe the study's limitations, are the conclusions supported by the results?

Critical appraisal of a published paper or report of a study

1 The aim(s) and /or objective(s) of the study should be stated clearly.

- The aim should state the purpose of the study succinctly and specifically. It should be set in the context of information that is already known from previously published literature.
- The reasons for, and need to carry out, the study should be justified in the introduction of the paper.
- There should be a clear route built up from the aim to the conclusion flowing from the explanation of why a particular study design, population and setting were selected, to the results reported, the discussion and interpretation, and final conclusion(s).

2 The methodology should be appropriate for the aim(s) of the study.

- Quantitative and qualitative design techniques are complementary. A good quantitative survey will be based on prior qualitative work to determine what are appropriate questions to ask in the questionnaire or interview schedule. A randomised controlled trial may be a gold standard quantitative study design, but a qualitative method will most probably be needed to report people's observations, reflections and judgements.
- As a generalisation, prospective recording is more likely to be accurate than retrospective recall.
- A sample of a population should be selected for study which is as representative as possible of the whole population.
- A setting should be chosen for a study which is as representative as possible of the setting of the total population to which the results of the study will be extrapolated.

- The sample size should be justified by a *power calculation* determined prior to starting the study based on the expected findings.
- There should be a method for increasing the response rate to as near as possible an ideal of 100% of the subjects included in the study.
- Details of any measurement or intervention should be as specific as possible, and transparently valid and reliable.
- A good study design will include a method to validate the questionnaire, rating scale or results obtained.
- It is always a bonus to see an original questionnaire, even if only in an abbreviated form, to be able to judge for yourself the validity of the questions used in the study.
- The statistical methods should be described so that when the results are reported readers can check the statistical calculations and understand how the results were derived from the original data, if they wish.

3   The results should be robust, justified and related to the objectives of the study.

- The results should be simple to understand. It should be obvious where the results have come from and they should not seem to have been plucked out of thin air. Graphs and tables help to avoid strings of numbers and percentages.
- Statistically significant results should be presented in a conventional way or explained with full references if less well-known statistical tests are used.
- Percentages should normally add up to 100% and if they do not there should be some explanation to account for the missing numbers. It should be clear where and whether subjects have not sent back the questionnaire, have left a particular question blank or given a 'don't know' response.
- If the results obtained from the subjects are fairly crude, such as when people are asked to estimate their answers or recall happenings in the distant past, the result should be given as whole numbers or to one decimal place, rather than to several decimal places, which might look more scientific to the casual reader.
- The written contents of a research paper should be in their correct places. Bits of method should not crop up afresh in the results, nor should discussion be interspersed in the results. The flow of the paper should be logical and build up to a justifiable conclusion. Anything otherwise is confusion and muddle.
- A low response rate may mean that the results from the sample of the population studied are not likely to be representative of the whole population. The further you regress from a 100% response rate the more likely it is that you have missed people or things that would give

your results a different slant. As a very rough guide, a response rate of 70% seems generally to be regarded as reasonable for a topic where the results are not going to have dire consequences if they are wrong. But if the study was a trial of drug therapy where people's lives might be at stake if the research results and conclusions were wrong, anything less than a 100% response rate might be unacceptable.

4 Any biases in the design and execution of the study should be minimised and their likely influences acknowledged and explained.

- Good response rates are important because responders may have different characteristics from those of non-responders.
- There may be confounding factors present. These are so-far undetected influences that were not measured or recorded in the course of the study, which were actually wholly or partly responsible for causing the changes or results reported. There are often cultural changes with time outside the study and beyond the control of those undertaking the investigation. For instance, if a famous celebrity claimed benefits for a new treatment that was being studied, many more people would suddenly believe they had received the same benefits and the outcomes being studied at that time would be distorted. Opting for *randomised controlled trials* avoids the influence of confounding factors.
- The potential and actual biases of the study should be openly described and their likely effects discussed in the Discussion section of the paper. Readers should then be able to make up their own minds about the relative importance of each bias on the results and how much the biases prejudice the extrapolation of the results to the readers' own situations.

5 Is the conclusion valid?

- The conclusion is often found in the Discussion section of a paper when there is no separate Conclusion section.
- The conclusions of the results should not hinge on probability test results. The significance of the results claimed should make sense from clinical and common sense perspectives too. For example, an intervention might claim that it is significantly better than another at increasing small children's height by 0.1 inches. But if, clinically, this difference is inconsequential, then the benefits of the treatment claiming to be superior are not proven by the positive significant result.
- The conclusion(s) should not make any claims that have not been justified previously in the report of the study.
- No new information should suddenly crop up in the conclusions that was not previously cited in the Method, Results or any other section.

- It should be clear what the main findings mean and the implications for current practice or future developments.
- The results of the current study should be compared and contrasted with others reported elsewhere, and any discrepancies interpreted and discussed.

6   Are there any other concerns about the study?

- Conflicts of interest should be stated, such as the sponsorship of the study by a manufacturer of the medication tested in the study.
- Look for any omissions in any section of the report. Think whether the implications from any contrary results seem to have been considered in full or glossed over.

Examples

Critically appraise this example – a summary report of a research study.

1 An investigation of the use of sunscreens in the United Kingdom

Summary

Aim: To investigate the use of sunscreens in children.

Method: A postal questionnaire was sent out to all 942 members of Women's Institutes throughout the Scottish Isles, asking them about the frequency of the use of high-factor sunscreens applied to their children (please contact the author for a copy of the questionnaire). Questionnaires were anonymous to ensure confidentiality. An article was placed in the Women's Institute newsletter to prompt non-responders.

Results: 356 women replied (85% response rate; average age $56 \pm SD$ 16.4298 years). 290 stated that they bought factor 10 or higher sunscreen. 89 preferred the scent-free version ($p < 0.1$). 350 women thought that the government should subsidise the cost of sunscreens as they were too expensive ($p < 0.0001$). The presence of a melanoma should be treated as a criminal offence and the sufferer fined for not having used sufficient sunscreen, as a contribution to the costs of the ensuing NHS treatment.

Conclusion: If the government were to subsidise the cost of buying high-factor sunscreens, uptake would be increased and the frequency of melanomas or other skin cancers would fall.

Source of funding: Nibblea Suncreams.

Conflict of interest: None.

Chambers R. *J Evidence-Based Spoof* 1998; **3**: 12.

Consider the following challenges

Write down your answers then read the author's opinion below:

1 Are the aim(s) and/or objective(s) of the study clearly stated?
2 Is the methodology appropriate for the aim(s) of the study?
3 Do the results relate to the aims(s) and/or objective(s) of the study? Are the results robust and justified?
4 Are there any biases in the design and execution of the study?
5 Is the conclusion valid?
6 Are there any other concerns about the study?

Critique of the summary report: use of sunscreens in the United Kingdom

1 Are the aim(s) and/or objective(s) of the study clearly stated?

The aim is not very specific. If the focus of the conclusion on cost of sunscreens and the impact of sunscreens on the frequency of cancers was intended as the purpose of the study then the aim has been expressed incorrectly.

2 Is the methodology appropriate for the aim(s) of the study?

No, no, no! There is already confusion as the aim and conclusions are so far apart, but working on the premise of the aim stated in the summary of the study given:

- the population chosen for study is inappropriate as children of Women's Institute members probably range in age from 1 to 60 years old; this can be deduced from the subject's average age being 56 years and the standard deviation (SD) of 16.4 years, indicating that about two-thirds of the population studied are between ca. 40 and 72 years (that is, 56 − 16.4 years = ~ 40 years to 56 + 16.4 years = 72 years)
- the Scottish Isles setting is in a part of the United Kingdom that would be expected to have relatively low amounts and strength of ultraviolet rays, and results from this setting cannot necessarily be generalised elsewhere
- members of Women's Institutes living in the Scottish Isles while the study was in progress had not necessarily lived there all their lives; so if the geographical area was important the mothers do not have uniform histories of where they lived when younger, and their children may have lived apart from their mothers at any time previously
- the age range of the children means that some mothers' reports will relate to children under the age of 18 years currently receiving modern types of high-factor sunscreens, and others will relate to middle-aged children who may or may not have had old-fashioned creams applied a

varying number of years previously; high-factor sunscreens did not exist at the time the study began
- there is no logic in choosing Women's Institute members as the population group to be studied – it may introduce a further bias if it were shown that members were more likely to be part of a more affluent section of society than the population as a whole and therefore more likely to take holidays abroad where the sunshine was more powerful and potentially damaging
- mothers' recall of the frequency of use of suncreams applied to children up to 50 years before is unlikely to be accurate
- anonymous questionnaires that do not bear a code number make chasing up of individual non-respondents impossible – an article placed in a newsletter is unlikely to be an effective method of encouraging non-responders to reply.

3   Do the results relate to the aim(s) and/or objective(s) of the study? Are the results robust and justified?

It is obvious that the results are inaccurate and meaningless. Also:

- the response rate was very low at 38% (356/942), not 85% as stated
- the results, such as the information about costs of sunscreens, are not related to the data that would have arisen from the study method described
- it is ridiculous to give the standard deviation (SD) to four decimal places when the average age is given as a whole number
- a probability of < 0.1 is not significant and no such conclusions can be drawn about a proportion of the population studied preferring the scent-free version
- results should be factual and not offer interpretations as here, where the government is encouraged to treat the presence of melanomas as a criminal offence
- the results cannot be generalised.

4   Are there any biases in the design and execution of the study?

The study is riddled with biases from start to finish. Many have been described already, such as:

- the nature of the population
- that retrospective recall of information is likely to be poor
- the poor response rate
- the changing nature of commercially available sunscreens over time throughout the study
- the fact that the conclusion does not relate to the rest of the study, which implies that the whole purpose of the study may have been to show that

sunscreens should be subsidised and that the design and reporting of the study might be biased to that end.

5 Is the conclusion valid?

No it is not. It does not follow from the rest of the report and is not related to the original aim.

6 Are there are any other concerns about the study?

Although the author of this report states that there was no conflict of interest, the sponsorship of the study by a manufacturer of suncreams should alert readers to scrutinise the report even more carefully than usual for possible biases.

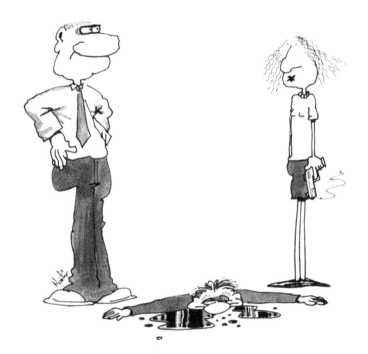

Remember that sometimes the evidence can be misleading.

2 Critically appraise this second example – why do teenagers become pregnant?

Answer the following challenges, as before – write down your answers then read the author's opinion:

1   are the aim(s) and/or objective(s) of the study clearly stated?
2   is the methodology appropriate for the aim(s) of the study?
3   do the results relate to the aim(s) and/or objective(s) of the study? Are the results robust and justified?
4   are there any biases in the design and execution of the study?
5   is the conclusion valid?
6   are there any other concerns about the study?

The following report concerns a real study carried out by one of the authors with colleagues, but the study design, findings and conclusions have been intentionally adulterated with apparent poor practice and mistakes to illustrate the learning points. All of the faults described below frequently appear in published papers, although not usually in such quantity and to such an exaggerated extent. The subsequent critique picks out main points and is not intended to be comprehensive – you will note more errors and poor research practice as you study the following section yourself.

Report: why do teenagers become pregnant?

Introduction: Nine out of 10 teenage mothers in one survey reported that their pregnancies were unplanned.[32] Most of these had not used contraception because sexual intercourse had been 'unexpected'. The younger the girl at first intercourse, the sooner intercourse had occurred in the relationship in one study of pregnant teenagers.[33] Many had not sought formal advice about contraception from either family planning clinics or general practitioners because they thought it was illegal for those under 16 years of age to obtain contraceptives or that their parents must be told, or because they felt embarrassed. Pearson et al.[34] reported that three-fifths of a cohort of pregnant teenagers had used condoms which had apparently leaked, split or come off.

About a fifth of women aged 16 to 49 years in England who require contraception go to family planning clinics and most of the rest go to general practitioners. The proportion of teenagers aged under 16 years who visit family planning clinics for contraception has increased over the last 20 years and it is estimated that in 1999–2000 about 43 000 females aged 15 years attended (about 14% of the population aged 15 years), and 25 000 girls aged under 15 years (about 4% of the population aged 13 to 14 years old). The proportion of women aged 16 to 19 years old who attended family planning clinics in 1999–2000 was 23%.

Aim: This study set out to determine reasons why teenagers become pregnant.

Method: A questionnaire was devised to enquire about the circumstances and reasons why teenagers became pregnant, their past use of contraceptives, their knowledge about contraceptives, possible exposure to HIV and other sexually transmitted diseases, and their smoking status. Teenagers were also asked if they had received advice about their future contraceptive needs.

Midwifery and ward staff working on the maternity and gynaecology wards of one general hospital administered questionnaires to teenage patients aged 19 years and under during a three-month period. The research nurse visited each ward every week to collect the completed questionnaires.

Data from the questionnaires was analysed using the statistical package SPSS.

Results: There were 113 live births to teenagers and 57 teenagers had a termination of pregnancy during the 12-week study period. Seventy-one of the 113 teenage in-patients completed questionnaires about the contraceptive services they had received whilst on the ward, and reasons why they had become pregnant. Seventeen of the 57 teenagers who had a termination of pregnancy completed questionnaires too; one other patient who had a termination refused to complete a questionnaire. Ward staff told the research nurse that they had been 'too busy' to remember to administer questionnaires to all teenagers in their care.

Seventeen subjects completed their questionnaires within one day of giving birth, 29 between one and two days and 25 more than two days after delivery. Those who had terminations responded before being discharged later the same day.

The most common reason, given by 34% of teenagers, for becoming pregnant was that no contraception had been used. A third had intended to become pregnant. Ten per cent had forgotten to take their contraceptive pills, one patient reported failure of emergency contraception pills taken correctly and two patients had become pregnant whilst taking antibiotics in addition to the contraceptive pill. The rest described using condoms which had burst during sexual intercourse.

There was a significant difference between the reasons given for becoming pregnant by those who had a live birth, and by those who had had a termination, in that those who had given birth were significantly more likely to have planned their pregnancy (p < 0.0001).

Table 1: Reasons for becoming pregnant given by teenagers who have had a live birth or termination of pregnancy

Reasons for pregnancy	Teenagers who have had live birth or termination (n = 88)
Planned	24
Forgot to take oral contraceptive pill	9
Condom burst	13
Condom slipped off	2
Failure of emergency contraception	4
Took antibiotics whilst on oral contraceptive pill	2
Multifactorial	1
Did not use contraception	39

Table 2: Midwives' perceptions about extent of contraceptive help given

Extent of help given	Teenagers who have had live birth or termination (n = 88)
'Learnt all they needed to know'	62
Time for questions limited	21
Did not want contraceptive advice	2
Family planning leaflets given	74
No family planning leaflets given	3
Did not want family planning leaflets	6

Discussion: This study involved a wide range of teenagers with different experiences – both those who had had a live birth and those who had had a termination; so results can be generalised to teenagers in general.

There was a perception gap between midwives and other hospital staff believing that contraceptive advice had been given whilst on the ward and teenage patients reporting that they had received it. It may be that improved procedures in the provision of contraceptive advice should be developed so that the advice given has more impact on these young patients.

Teenagers viewed both family planning clinics and general practitioners' surgeries as important providers of contraceptive services. Young persons' clinics were not well known to these subjects.

A substantial proportion of pregnant teenagers had not used any form of contraception. This was probably because they had been unable to obtain the right help at the right time.

Condom failures were commonly blamed for unplanned pregnancies, usually because they burst; this should be investigated further to find out if bursting is due to inadequate fitting techniques or poor manufacture.

Conclusions: Teenagers who have just had a termination are ideally placed to receive contraceptive advice as they are 'trapped' in their hospital bed and should be motivated by not wanting to have another termination in the future.

Condoms should be more durable and much stronger so that they do not burst as easily.

The midwives in this study were lazy in that they only administered questionnaires to just over half the teenage patient subjects.

Teenagers find family planning leaflets very useful for giving them advice about future contraceptive needs.

Critique of the report: Why do teenagers become pregnant?

1 Are the aim(s) and/or objective(s) of the study clearly stated?
   The aim given is narrower than some of the other issues covered in the study. The bulk of the material given in the Introduction concerns teenagers' usage rates of family planning clinics and sources of contraceptive provision, rather than literature focused on reasons for teenagers becoming pregnant. In the Method section, enquiry was made about sexually transmitted diseases; and in the results and discussion sections, midwives reported whether they had provided contraceptive advice whilst teenagers were inpatients. The aim and objectives should cover the scope of the study.
2 Is the methodology appropriate for the aim(s) of the study?
   • Interviews might have been more appropriate than an administered questionnaire to ensure that the interviewees understood the questions and in order to elicit sensitive information.
   • The study was conducted in only one location whereas the aim of the study implies that the findings to the question being asked should be generalisable and there is no attempt to consider the extent to which the location studied is representative of England/UK/western world or whatever was intended.
   • The questionnaire should include young people's perspectives of their concerns and issues; so the method could have involved preliminary work with young people to gather their views and compose the questionnaire using their language and including their issues and priorities.
   • There was no power calculation or indication of whether 88 subjects was a valid number to study and likely to give a reliable result.
   • There was no mention of ethical approval or research governance agreement having been gained, or subjects giving informed consent before participating in the study.
   • Those administering the questionnaire (midwives and other ward staff) did not appear to be sufficiently involved in the research process and thus they often 'forgot' to administer the questionnaire to teenage subjects. It may also be that different midwives and other staff did not

administer the questionnaire in an impartial way and biased the responses; and that there was variability between midwives and other ward staff in the way that questionnaires were administered.

- Subjects responded at varying times after delivery or termination, and this may have given them unequal opportunities for having received contraceptive advice whilst on the ward.

3 Do the results relate to the aim(s) and objective(s) of the study? Are the results robust and justified?

- The results from teenagers who had given birth, and those who had had a termination, should not have been added together as a joint result, without much more detailed analysis to check if the characteristics of both groups were so similar that adding their results together was justified. In this case, it seems the two groups of teenagers are very different and should be considered separately.
- There is an error in the figures in Table 1, which do not add up to the number of subjects (n = 88). There are no figures or indication if there were non-respondents.
- There is a reference to SPSS but no mention of what statistical test was used to calculate the probability result.
- In Table 2 it is not clear if there were any non-respondents, and readers cannot check for themselves as midwife respondents appear able to give more than one answer, although this is not clear.
- The reports of the reasons for becoming pregnant are a mixture of percentages and actual numbers, so the actual results are omitted.
- There is too little information about the non-respondents and reasons for non-response.
- As noted before, results are given that are outside the scope of the given aim. Some results are given for which there was nothing in the method section about how that information was collected, e.g. about midwives being asked for their perceptions of the extent of contraceptive help provided to teenage in-patients. Some information was described as being collected in the method (e.g. about sexually transmitted diseases), but for which no results are given. Some information is given in the discussion (e.g. reference to teenagers' views about contraceptive help received) which does not appear in the results section.

4 Are there any biases in the design and execution of the study?

- The focus of the introduction on usage of family planning clinics and accidents with condoms, to the exclusion of literature reporting other reasons for teenagers becoming pregnant, seems to reflect a bias running through the whole study.
- There is not enough information about the subjects to understand if they are representative of teenagers in general. The study is confined to one general hospital somewhere in England and may not be generalisable to

the general population of teenagers in the rest of England and beyond. So the method might have included comparison between different geographic locations, or collected more data about the socio-economic characteristics or educational attainment, etc. of subjects and compared those figures with the population at which the study was aimed.

- The midwives and other ward staff who administered the questionnaires might have influenced the teenagers' completion of the questionnaires if they did not value the study and made known their feelings that it was a waste of time, or if the youngsters thought that individual midwives would see their answers and were reluctant to displease the staff.

- The timing of the study might have meant that recent emotional and physical experiences of a live birth or termination affected the answers given by the teenage respondents.

5   Are the conclusions valid?

- Many of the conclusions are not justified by the results obtained. For instance, although 'burst' condoms was commonly reported, that may have been an excuse teenagers used rather than admit they had neglected to use contraception in the heat of the moment, or poor technique might have been the real reason for condoms failing. Extrapolating from the results to recommend that condoms be manufactured to be more durable is not supported by the findings of the study.

- The conclusion that immediately after a termination is an ideal time to provide contraceptive help seems to have originated from the beliefs and preferences of the authors of the study rather than information gathered during the research process.

- No information was gathered as to the workload of midwives on the wards. The supposition that they were 'lazy' because they did not prioritise administering questionnaires from the study in their everyday practice is a subjective conclusion of the authors of the study that was not tested for, nor is it borne out by the findings.

- Teenagers were not questioned about how useful they found the information in the family planning leaflets they were given, according to the method that is described. It cannot be concluded that just because they received contraceptive literature they found it useful.

6   Are there any other concerns about the study?

- The question posed 'Why do teenagers become pregnant?' is a very widely-based question that will have a multifactorial answer and cannot be answered in a healthcare setting alone – it should include social, educational and parenting elements at least.

- Statistics are cited in the Introduction but no reference is given.

- The timing does not seem appropriate for obtaining reliable and valid information to answer this question, coming as it does immediately after emotionally traumatic events such as giving birth or having a termination.

- There is no mention of consumer involvement in the form of teenagers themselves, in planning, undertaking or interpreting the results of this study.

Critical appraisal of a qualitative research paper

Although qualitative research is not part of the hierarchy of evidence, it can provide a useful source of evidence. Qualitative research has been used extensively in the fields of nursing and midwifery, allied health professionals (AHPs), mental health and the evaluation of the health service. Indeed, many midwives and AHPs searching for evidence in respect of their disciplines may find that while no quantitative research has been undertaken, there may be a number of published qualitative studies. Thus, it is essential that you are able to make a judgement about the quality of these types of studies as well. The following checklist and reminders about features you should consider is modified from Greenhalgh and Taylor (1997).[35]

1 Did the paper address an important clinical problem? Was the research question clearly formulated and defined?
   There should be a clear statement about why the research was done and the research question that was addressed.

2 Is a qualitative approach the best method of answering this research question?
   Qualitative research is useful for exploring beliefs, feelings and perceptions; for gaining a deeper understanding of an area; for exploring situations where little is known; for exploring sensitive issues; for gaining the 'whole picture'; and for allowing participants to speak for themselves. If this is what is being done, then a qualitative approach is almost certainly best. But think whether a quantitative approach, such as a randomised controlled trial (RCT), would have been more appropriate.

3 Is the setting/context for the research clear? How were the subjects selected? Is the sampling strategy described in detail? Is this strategy justified?
   Qualitative research is about exploring the beliefs and gaining a deeper understanding of the experiences of a particular group of people or individuals. The sample is therefore selected in order to include people from these groups. That is, people are chosen because they are part of that group, rather than being chosen at random or to represent the 'average' view.

4 Have the researcher's perspective, beliefs, experiences and background been taken into account?
   'Researcher' or 'observer' bias is important in qualitative research as the interviewer's background, knowledge, experience, beliefs, etc., may have an influence on the results of semi-structured interviews and focus groups. It is impossible to eliminate researcher bias, so the authors should address this problem by discussing the researcher's perspective and how this might have influenced the interpretation of the results.

5 What data collection methods were used and are these described in detail?
   Rigorous reporting of methods in articles about qualitative research is particularly important, as each study is unique in design and analysis. The methods tell the 'story' that is needed to interpret the results. Hoddinott and Pill (1997) suggest that you should ask the following questions:

   - *are the researchers' roles and qualifications clear?*
   - *are interviewer details given?*
   - *is the paper explicit about how respondents were recruited, who recruited them and how the research was explained to them?*
   - *is it explicit about whether the interviewer was known to the respondents and how they were introduced?*
   - *is the interview setting clearly stated?*
   - *were methodological issues about the influence of the interviewer on the data addressed?*

6 What methods were used to analyse the data? What quality control measures were implemented? Was an attempt made to test the validity of the results? Was an attempt made to test the reliability of the results?
   There are various different methods of analysing qualitative data, e.g. content analysis and grounded theory. You should look for evidence that the researcher has analysed the data in a systematic way. Do the authors state that the data, e.g. transcripts, field notes or audio tapes, are available for independent review? The authors should have looked for cases which contradict the developing theories. The data should have been independently analysed by another researcher or a second researcher should have repeated the analysis.

7 Are the results credible? Are the findings clinically important?
   Use your common sense and ask 'Do the results seem sensible and believable? Will they matter in practice?' You should also look at whether the authors present sufficient original data, e.g. verbatim quotes, and whether these are indexed to subjects so that they could be traced back and checked.

8 What conclusions were made? Are the conclusions justified by the results?
   In qualitative research the results and the discussion are not separate as in quantitative research, as the results are an interpretation of the data. You can look

for evidence that the conclusions are 'grounded in evidence', i.e. that they flow from the findings, how comprehensible the explanations are, how well the analysis explains why people behave in the way they do, and how well the explanation fits with what is already known.

9　Can the findings be transferred to other clinical settings?
　　Qualitative research is often criticised for only being applicable to the setting in which it was conducted. However, if true theoretical sampling rather than simply convenience sampling has been used, then the results are likely to be more transferable.

The checklist outlined above is not as all-encompassing or universally applicable as a checklist for critically appraising quantitative research, as qualitative research is 'by its very nature, non-standard, unconfined, and dependent on the subjective experience of both the researcher and the researched'.[35] This checklist sets some useful ground rules which may be enhanced by information given in other sources.[36,37]

Critically appraise a published paper

Now that you have learned to critically appraise a research report, try your hand at appraising a published paper. Refer back to the explanations about randomised controlled trials, probability, confidence limits or other scientific terms described in the earlier text if necessary. The same rules apply for carrying out a survey of all research about a topic as for individual research papers. The specific question being addressed must be stated explicitly, the subject population (relevant research reports) identified and accessed, appropriate information obtained in an unbiased fashion (by using specific criteria to identify which research reports should, and should not, be included in the review) and the final conclusions should relate to the evidence obtained from the research reports included in the publication related back to the primary survey question.

　Look particularly for information in the publication to reassure you of the following:

• The topic and purpose of the research are specified.
• The search methods used to find evidence relating to the question should be stated. The review of the literature should be comprehensive – reasonable efforts should have been made to identify and include relevant studies by consulting a range of databases and tracking down 'grey' material such as that in books, from conference proceedings, consensus statements or annual reports.

- The research included in the report should be relevant and appropriate to the main subject or issue being addressed.
- Only similar data have been combined from different studies with similar subject characteristics, circumstances and methodologies. The methods used to combine the findings of the studies included in the research publication should be stated.
- There should be enough details about the subjects, populations, settings and other important factors for you to be able to decide whether the report's results and conclusions will be relevant to your particular circumstances.
- The criteria used to define whether or not a study was included in the overview should be stated clearly in the Methods section. The researchers should have adhered to those explicit inclusion criteria, avoiding any bias in their method of selection.
- The results should be presented clearly in a scientific way. The results should be understandable, numbers in tables should add up, and it should be obvious how any analyses were derived.
- The authors should describe how the quality of the papers was assessed – how many people assessed each paper, whether they were blinded to other researchers' opinions, what criteria of quality were used, whether these criteria were valid, reliable and reproducible, and whether they adhered to the criteria.
- The results should be relevant to the declared aim of the research report.
- The results should be generalisable – the significance of different biases should be considered and their implications discussed. The author(s) should give a critical analysis of the scientific rigour of the studies in the report, with all interpretative remarks being justified.
- The results should be comprehensive. Negative as well as positive findings in the different studies should be described. The range of confidence limits gives more information than a mere probability statistic.
- The conclusions should be based on an overview of the data and/or analyses of all the studies included in the report.
- The outcomes should indicate clearly any modifications that should be made to future healthcare practice based on the evidence presented in the report.

If you want to practise your critical appraisal skills obtain a copy of the following publication:

- Hannah M, Hannah W, Hewson S, Hodnett E *et al.* Planned caesarean section versus planned vaginal birth for breech presentation at term: a randomised multicentre trial. *The Lancet* 2000; **357**: 1375–83.

Read through the article first to get a feel for it. Then read it again conscientiously, absorbing the details and making notes as ideas and concerns come to mind. Now use the information given above, writing down your answers. The whole critical appraisal exercise should take you about three hours. Turn over and read how *we* reviewed this journal paper.

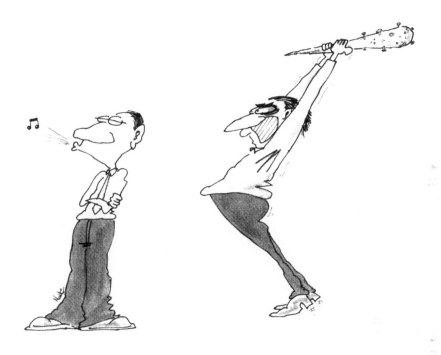

It may be hard to convince your colleagues even when you've got the evidence.

Our review of Hannah M, Hannah W, Hewson S *et al*. Planned caesarean section versus planned vaginal birth for breech presentation at term.[38]

The following critique is a summary based on the published opinion of Glezerman[39] and views of the authors of this book. It is difficult to dissociate fact and interpretation in the critical appraisal of published papers and as several of the comments that follow are a matter of interpretation and opinion, you may well disagree with our critique. Many of the weaknesses of the paper that we highlight have already been recognised by the original researchers and midwifery community.[40,41] This study has therefore been selected as one from which we can all learn.

Are the topic and purpose of the study clearly specified?

Yes, the aim was to determine whether there are benefits from planned caesarean section compared with planned vaginal delivery for breech presentation at term.

What was the overall conclusion of the study?

The Term Breech Trial study[38] concluded that delivery by planned caesarean section has substantially better outcomes for the singleton foetus in the breech presentation at term than for planned vaginal delivery. But planned caesarean section was only an advantage if preterm caesarean section was performed before or during early labour. For those women for whom caesarean section was performed during active labour, it appeared that there was only a borderline difference in perinatal outcome.

How precise are the results?

Serious concerns have been voiced as to the study design, methods and conclusions.[39] For instance, there was substantial variation in the standards of care provided between institutions participating in the research study; with many having inadequate methods of ante partum and intra partum foetal assessment. A large proportion of women were recruited late into the study during active labour. In many cases of planned vaginal delivery studied, attending clinicians did not have adequate expertise.

Some of the major concerns about the overall adherence of the research undertaken in relation to the study criteria are:

- application of inclusion criteria
  In more than one third of women, no imaging studies were performed to ascertain whether hyperextension of the foetal head was present. Yet hyperextension of the foetal head is a widely accepted contraindication for vaginal delivery and cannot be fully assessed by clinical examination alone.[39]

  Although the research design stated that only live singleton foetuses at term were to be included in the study, there were two sets of twins, one case of anencephalus and two stillbirths among the perinatal deaths reported.[39]

  In general, most clinicians would avoid performing vaginal deliveries with large babies with breech presentation. But in this study, some foetuses had a birth weight greater than 4000g in the planned vaginal delivery group.[39]
- differences in the standards of care between participating study centres
  Study sites had different standards of care. A centre was classed as having a 'high' standard of care if 'caesarean section could be performed within 10 minutes, if there were the immediate availability of resuscitation by providing oxygen through bag/mask or endotracheal intubation and positive pressure ventilation, and if there were personnel and infrastructure available to provide ventilation for greater than 24 hours.' A centre was classed as providing 'usual' standard of care if these criteria could not be met.[38] In the research study, one third of centres provided a high standard of care and two-thirds usual standard of care. So the perinatal outcomes from centres classed as delivering 'usual standard of care' cannot be generalised to the majority of maternity centres in the western world where their normal levels of care can be classified as being at the 'high' standard.[39]
- lack of clinicians with adequate expertise
  Twenty-two cases of perinatal death described in the study were attended by obstetricians in training or without experience or in one case a midwife without experience.[39]
- variation from best practice guidance
  Whilst accepted guidance in delivering a baby with vaginal breech presentation is to be 'hands off the breech', the approach used in this study varied and included 'gentle traction while encouraging the mother to push'.

Can the results be applied and generalised?

Glezerman has published a critical analysis of the perinatal mortality cases in the study which concludes that most cases of perinatal death were not related to the mode of delivery.

Concerns have been expressed as to whether women in the midst of labour are in a fit state to be able to give informed consent to be randomly assigned to various management approaches in a clinical trial.[39]

It is thought that there was improper randomisation of all eligible patients in this study which may have led to an unacceptable number of stillbirths, twins and other babies with intrauterine growth retardation and congenital malformations being included in the trial.[39]

Glezerman suggests that the Term Breech Trial[38] has been based on such serious methodological and clinical flaws that the results cannot be generalised.[39] Yet a recent survey carried out in more than 80 centres in 23 countries, concluded that the vast majority of maternity centres have completely abandoned planned vaginal breech delivery in favour of caesarean section[41] – seemingly a direct result of the original study.[38] Glezerman proposes that the recommendations from the Term Breech Trial[38] should be withdrawn. It seems that another trial needs to be undertaken to determine the safest mode of delivery for breech presentation with a revised clinical design and methodology compared to those adopted in the Term Breech Trial.

Stage 5

Apply the evidence

You have identified your problem, posed your question with help from colleagues at work, searched for the best available evidence, judged the quality of the evidence, weighed the relative importance of any conflicting results, applied the evidence theoretically to your own circumstances and situation, and now you should be ready to apply the evidence in practice.

Clinicians have expressed concern about the dangers of adhering blindly to evidence in practice, and fears that evidence-based practice might be regarded as the be-all and end-all as far as decisions about the cost-effective delivery of health services go. Clinical judgement and common sense must be paramount in keeping evidence in perspective. The information forming the 'evidence' may be irrelevant, incomplete or inaccurate, or the 'evidence' may simply not be applicable in the particular clinical circumstances in question. The NHS has a long way to go in accumulating a bank of good and reliable information about current clinical care and best practices.

Do not regard the evidence generated in randomised controlled trials as sacrosanct. They may provide the best sort of evidence for evaluating the benefits of alternative medications, but they are not necessarily the best way of identifying evidence for resolving more complex human health issues.

Evidence-based management has an even weaker information base than evidence-based clinical practice. It must be right to encourage practice managers and other health service managers to adopt a research culture with a questioning approach. This will encourage them to reflect about what is happening, how and why, and to compare management practices.

So bear all this in mind as you think about applying the evidence you have gained from your search to your particular clinical situation. You may like to think of making changes from the perspective of an individual clinician, a practice or unit, or a primary care organisation or hospital trust.

Diary of your progress in searching for evidence

Complete this summary of progress to date and your action plan for how you propose to introduce any changes in your working practices.

Write a summary of:

1 your problem (be as specific as possible so that you can measure the outcomes of any changes against this baseline position):

2 your question:

3 your search method – where you searched (databases, people):

4 the types of your best evidence (systematic review, randomised controlled trials, controlled trials, reports, conference proceedings, expert opinions):

5 ... give three titles of the most relevant and appropriate publications or sources that you found:

6 your conclusion(s) from the best evidence available in answer to your question:

7 the change(s) that you propose to make yourself or that others should make, as a result of the evidence you have obtained and the conclusion(s) you have drawn:

Action plan

People to whom you have fed back the results of the evidence:

Have you already written a timetabled action plan?   *Yes/No*

The baseline position:

Whom have you involved in discussions about the change(s) you propose?

Change(s) proposed:

People whom the proposed change(s) will affect:

Additional resources that will be required (people, premises, time, money, skills, etc.):

The timetable is:

Who will do what:

Advantages or health gains expected:

Disadvantages or losses (opportunity costs) that may happen:

How and when the changed situation will be monitored again:

Barriers to change

Once evidence has been gathered, projects have been completed and necessary changes discussed, there can still be many barriers to overcome before worthwhile changes can happen.

The King's Fund PACE[6] initiative identified the following barriers to change:

- others' lack of perception of the relevance of your proposed change (you should have realised this during your initial consultations with colleagues before you began)
- lack of resources to implement the change (time, staff, skills, equipment)
- short-term outlook of work colleagues
- conflicting priorities – without additional resources, changes have the potential to cause work overload or opportunity costs
- difficulties in measuring outcomes – it is difficult to find acceptable worthwhile health outcomes that are easily measured
- lack of necessary skills (forward planning is needed)
- no tradition of multidisciplinary working (this problem can probably only be surmounted with a culture change)
- limitations of research evidence on effectiveness (there is a lot more research about problems than there is about effective solutions)
- perverse incentives (a common flaw in the way the NHS functions)
- the intensity of others' contribution that is required (again consult early, get everyone on board and encourage everyone to 'own' your project).

And so ...

- anticipate the strength of evidence you will need to convince your colleagues that the efforts and costs of change will be worthwhile – to them and the patients. Do this through clinical governance – understand how to make clinical governance work for you in the next chapter.

Read more about the lessons to be learned in how to make successful changes happen.[6]

Box 1 gives an example of how research can be applied in practice, by training practitioners in new evidence-based approaches. The educational programme that was run as six updating skills workshops between 2002–2004, was derived from the randomised controlled trial described in the following publication: Andrews V, Thakar R, Sultan A, Kettle C. Can hands on perineal repair courses affect clinical practice? *British Journal of Midwifery* 2005: **13**(9): 562–5.

Box 1   An example of how research was put into practice: can hands-on perineal repair courses improve clinical practice?

Summary of evidence

Eighty five per cent of women who have a spontaneous vaginal birth will have some form of perineal repair and up to 69 % will need to have sutures. Most of the women will have perineal pain in the period immediately after delivery and about a fifth will continue to have long term problems, such as superficial

---

dyspareunia. A large randomised controlled trial provided evidence that the continuous technique should be used for repair of second degree tears and episiotomies, and that using the more rapidly absorbing polyglactin 910 compared with standard polyglactin 910 resulted in a greater than four fold reduction in the number of women requiring suture removal.

Educational programme

Six hands-on workshops were run to educate midwives and doctors in perineal anatomy and identification of obstetric anal sphincter injuries. The workshop also served to teach the participants to suture second degree tears using the continuous technique; 208 clinicians attended. This one day course comprised a series of lectures, video demonstrations and hands-on teaching using specifically designed suture foam pads and models. Practical hands-on skills taught included rectal examination, instrument handling, needle tip protection, suture technique and knot replacement. In order to evaluate a change in practice a self-administered questionnaire was completed prior to, and following, the workshop. The results in Tables 3 and 4 give the perceived responses from those participants who completed both pre-course and follow-up questionnaires.

Results

Table 3   Correct classification of anal sphincter trauma (n=149)

	Before course	After course
External anal sphincter (EAS) partially torn	114	127
EAS completely torn	105	126
Internal anal sphincter (IAS) exposed but not torn	94	122
IAS torn	67	100
Anal sphincter and mucosa torn	119	132

Table 4   Technique of performing perineal repair (n=135)

	Before course	After course
Continuous suture to the vagina	124	129
Continuous suture to the perineal muscles	43	114
Subcuticular suture to the skin	52	110

After the course the majority of participants had converted to the evidence-based practice approach and reported that they were using the continuous method of repair for vaginal mucosa, perineal muscle and skin.

Stage 6

What clinical governance means and how to put it into practice

Clinical governance is inclusive, making quality everyone's business, whether they are a doctor or a midwife, manager or member of the administrative staff, a patient or a strategic planner. We need to know where we are now and where we want to get to if we are to drive up standards of healthcare. Clinical effectiveness and clinical audit are central to this process.[42]

'Clinical governance is the framework through which organisations influence the informal psychology and social functioning of their staff. Its delivery will result in every clinical team putting quality at the heart of their moment to moment care of patients. ... Clinical governance ... enables the vocation and motivation of healthcare professionals and patients by giving their personal energy a voice: allowing them to meaningfully and continuously improve the culture they are part of. It encapsulates an organisation's statutory responsibility for the delivery of safe, high-quality patient care and it is the vehicle through which that accountable performance is made explicit.'[43]

Components of clinical governance

The components of clinical governance are well established. Bringing them together under the banner of clinical governance with explicit accountability for performance maintains quality in healthcare. The reception given to clinical governance ranges from an enthusiastic welcome to the cautious warning that innovations that improve quality may increase rather than decrease costs. Carefully evaluating your work and demonstrating subsequent improvements in patient care will enable you to form your own view about the place of clinical governance.

The following 14 themes are core components of professional and service development which, taken together, form a comprehensive approach to providing high-quality healthcare services and clinical governance. These are illustrated in the tree diagram:[42]

If you interweave these into your individual and workplace-based personal and professional development plans, you will have addressed the requirements for clinical governance at the same time.[44]

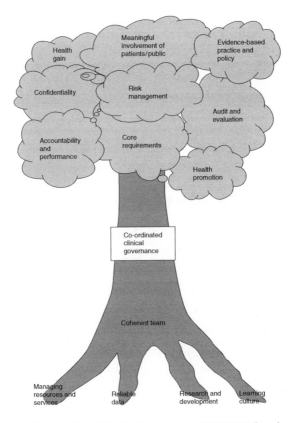

Figure 2: 'Routes' and branches of clinical governance (©2000 Chambers and Wakley).

1 **Learning culture**: in the practice, the primary care organisation, the trust and the NHS at large.
2 **Research and development culture**: throughout the health service.
3 **Reliable and accurate data**: in the practice, the primary care organisation and the NHS as a seamless whole.
4 **Well-managed resources and services**: as individuals, as a practice, as a primary care organisation or trust, across the NHS and in conjunction with social care and local authorities.
5 **Coherent team**: well-integrated teams within a practice, across a practice, in the primary care organisation or trust.
6 **Meaningful involvement of patients and the public**: in a practice or the NHS as a whole, including users, carers and the general population.

7 **Health gains**: activities to improve the health of patients in a practice, between practices, in the primary care organisation (PCO) or trust, and different geographical areas of the NHS.

8 **Confidentiality**: of information in consultations, in medical notes, between practitioners.

9 **Evidence-based practice and policy**: applying it in practice, in the primary care organisation or trust, in the district, across the NHS.

10 **Accountability and performance**: for standards, performance of individuals, the practice, primary care organisation or trust, health authority/board and the NHS, to the public and those in authority.

11 **Core requirements**: good fit with skill-mix and whether individuals are competent to do their jobs, communication, workforce numbers, morale at practice level, across the NHS.

12 **Health promotion**: for patients, the public, opportunistic and in general, targeting those with most needs.

13 **Audit and evaluation**: for instance, of changes, of individuals' and practices' performance, of the primary care organisation's or trust's achievements, of district services.

14 **Risk management**: pro-active review, follow-up, risk management, risk reduction.

The challenges to delivering clinical governance

Delivering high-quality healthcare with guaranteed minimum standards of care for users at all times, is a major challenge. At present the quality of healthcare is patchy and variable. We aren't very good at detecting underperformance and then taking the initiative and rectifying it at an early stage. The small number of clinicians who do underperform exert a disproportionately large effect on the public's confidence. Causes of underperformance in an individual might relate to a lack of knowledge or skills, poor attitudes or ill health. A lack of management capability is nearly always an important contributory factor to inadequate clinical services or the provision of healthcare.

We need to understand why variation exists and explore ways of reducing inequalities. Variation in the quality of healthcare provided is common – between different practices in the same locality, between staff of the same discipline working in the same practice or unit, between care given to some groups of the population rather than others. There may be up to four-fold differences in rates of referral to hospital for a particular condition, between one doctor and another, for example; some practices have attached social workers and community psychiatric nurses while others do not, for instance.

Good practice means understanding and managing risk – both clinical and organisational aspects. Integrating risk management into all that you do is one of the key steps in preserving patient safety.[45] Identifying new cases of important conditions such as diabetes and undertaking audit more systematically will reduce the risks of omission – in detection and clinical management. The common areas of risk in providing healthcare services are:

- out-of-date clinical practice – and insufficient investment in staff learning
- lack of continuity of care
- poor communication – in the organisation, between clinician and patient
- mistakes in patient care – known and unknown
- patient complaints and lack of response to complaints
- financial risk – insufficient resources
- concerns about reputation – of organisation or individuals
- low staff morale.

Clinical governance offers a co-ordinated approach to overcoming these areas of risk through a blend of clinical and organisational improvements to the quality of healthcare practice. Initiatives such as practice-based commissioning present risks for both trusts and practices. It adds complexity and requires sound governance and accountability.[46]

We need to agree on indicators of performance that are acceptable to clinicians and managers alike. It is often said that we tend to use outcomes that are the easiest to measure but which mean least in terms of the real quality of patient care.

Enhancing your personal and professional development

Education and training programmes should be relevant to service needs, whether at organisational or individual levels. Continuing professional development (CPD) programmes need to meet both the learning needs of individual health professionals and the wider service development needs of the NHS. You should no longer opt for CPD activities according to what you *want* to do, but rather, what you *need* to do. Clinical governance underpins professional and service development.[44]

Lifelong learning and CPD are integral to the concept of clinical governance and that includes everyone in a practice or department of a trust working towards agreed learning goals that are relevant to service development. Practitioners can review the balance between their own and NHS priorities at their annual appraisal. See Stage 7 to see how this will link with revalidation.

---

individual personal development plans
will feed into a
workplace- or practice-based personal and professional development plan
that will feed into
the organisation's business plan
all
underpinned by clinical governance[44]

Good morale and job satisfaction are prerequisites of learning and effective working, and should be nurtured by targeted personal and professional development plans. Clinical governance should be creating a culture and working environment where people thrive and feel fulfilled by their work.

1 How evidence-based care, clinical effectiveness and other components of clinical governance fit together: the practitioner's or the unit's perspective[42]

Learning culture

You cannot learn about the cultural changes needed for providing multidisciplinary, team-based healthcare in the modern health service by sitting passively in a lecture. You need to experience the learning and interact with others who will be part of that new culture. Historically, health professionals have been keener to attend lectures than interactive educational activities such as organised small group sessions or informal teaching in their workplaces.

The type or mode of education and training should be relevant to the topic of the learning and the characteristics or circumstances of the 'students'.

Maximising learning about the new requirements of the NHS will involve:

- setting up in-house formal and informal education and training opportunities
- everyone creating personal development plans that incorporate all modes of learning: reading and reflecting, shadowing others, small group discussions, online materials, as well as lectures and seminars
- a practice- or directorate-wide approach to a topic so that a portfolio of experience is built up to which everyone contributes – useful for revalidation and re-registration of team members' professional qualifications.

> Using a questionnaire is full of pitfalls and it is one of the most difficult techniques for gaining a true or valid answer to the question posed.

Applying research and development in practice

One of the most common research and development activities undertaken by health professionals is a questionnaire survey of their patients. A poorly designed patient satisfaction survey will give you meaningless results so that all the time and effort spent on the satisfaction survey is wasted, and changes made as a result of such a survey still do not satisfy the patient population. Patient satisfaction questionnaires are commonly used in hospital and general practice, as a hybrid of research and audit. Novices may mistakenly believe that undertaking a questionnaire survey is one of the simplest and easiest methods.

To try and ensure that a patient satisfaction survey is a meaningful exercise:

- use a questionnaire that has been tried and tested by someone else and is valid for your workplace setting
- make sure that the questions are relevant and appropriate to the purpose of the enquiry
- use questions which have an easily answered format with simple choices of response
- use appropriate language likely to be understood by all respondents, with translations into other languages if there are non-English speakers in your target population
- avoid leading questions that imply you are expecting a particular answer, otherwise respondents will tend to give the answer implied as being the 'right' one because they want to please you
- pilot your draft questionnaire to detect problems with your questions or method.

Reliable and accurate data

Clinicians, patients and administrators need reliable and accurate data to connect individuals or their healthcare records to other knowledge that is relevant to the care of the patient.

Set standards for a general practice:

- summarise medical records; within a specified time period for records of new patients
- review dates for checks on medication; with audit in place to monitor standards adhered to and plan for underperformance if necessary
- establish chronic disease registers and keep them updated
- use computers for diagnostic recording
- record information from external sources – hospital, other organisations – relevant to individual patients or the practice as a whole.

Think of the data you should collect about your or others' performance too. There should be 'effective systems in place to give early warning of any failure or potential failure in clinical performance ....'[47]

Well-managed resources and services

The things you need to achieve best practice should be in the right place at the right time and working correctly every time.

Set standards in your workplace for:

- access to premises and availability of services for people with special needs, such as those with sensory and visual impairments
- provision of routine and urgent appointments
- access to and provision for referral for investigation or treatment
- pro-active monitoring of chronic illness and disability
- alternatives to face-to-face consultations
- consultation length.

Primary care services to which the public requires access are: information, advice, triage and treatment, continuity of care, personal care and other services. Minimising inequalities and the outcomes of new skill-mix models are two prime concerns at the heart of considerations about access and evaluating standards, especially with regard to:

- level of access versus quality of care received
- access for those who demand more versus equity of access for all based on need
- an impersonal service versus continuity of care versus personal care

- a demand-led (by patients) service versus a service that is prioritised or rationed
- access to one particular member of the care team, first or above others
- substitution of, or delegation to, staff members.

Systems should be designed to prevent and detect errors. So keep systems simple and sensible, and inform everyone how systems operate so that they are less likely to bypass the system or make errors.

Concentrate on ensuring that your systems are designed to deliver care that is:

- safe
- effective
- accessible
- reliable
- efficient
- timely
- equitable
- patient-centred.[48]

Coherent teamwork

Teams produce better patient care than single practitioners operating in a fragmented way. Effective teams make the most of the different contributions of individual clinical disciplines in delivering patient care. The characteristics of effective teams are:

- shared ownership of a common purpose
- clear goals for the contributions each discipline makes
- open communication between team members
- opportunities offered for team members to enhance their skills.

A team approach helps different team members adopt an evidence-based approach to patient care, by having to justify their approach to the rest of the team.[49]

The experiences of teamwork on the Wirral[49]

The team was composed by a family support worker employed by the voluntary sector joining a community psychiatric nursing team. They found that the factors that helped the team to work well were:

- that each member of the team had a separate function
- joint training which cemented the team, although obstacles from different employer arrangements had to be overcome
- interdisciplinary differences of opinion about patient care being welcomed as a way of increasing debate and generating a wider range of options for care.

Meaningful involvement of patients and the public

The terms 'user' and 'public' are employed here to include patients or users, carers, non-users of services, the local community, a particular subgroup of the population and the general public.

If user involvement and public participation are done well they should result in:

- reductions in health inequalities
- better outcomes of individual care
- better health for the population
- better quality and more locally responsive services
- greater ownership of health services
- a better understanding of why and how local services need to be changed and developed.

Public participation may be organised at five levels and you should aim for true participation at the fifth level whenever possible:[50]

- **Level 1**: information exchange
- **Level 2**: consultation: the public and patients express their views but the consultant makes the decisions
- **Level 3**: support: the public decides what to do and others support them in doing it
- **Level 4**: deciding together: thinking and planning together
- **Level 5**: acting together: putting plans into action together.

A meaningful public consultation involves the exchange of information between the healthcare providers and the general public, obtaining a representative opinion as a result that feeds into the local decision-making process of healthcare services or whoever is sponsoring the consultation.

How to go about undertaking meaningful consultation[51]

Be clear about:

- the purpose of the exercise: is it important and is it necessary?
- the type and identity of the population to whom the purpose relates
- how to reach and engage the target population
- the extent and mode of information exchange required prior to consultation
- the implications of the methods you employ in the consultation – what outputs you expect from the consultation
- how you will act on the results of the consultation
- how you will feed back the outcome of the consultation exercise
- how you will evaluate the consultation exercise.

You may have to trade off a relatively cheaper method of consultation that engages with fewer people or with a less representative section of the population subgroup; if you do, you will need to understand what biases are arising and make allowances for those biases when you interpret the results of the consultation.

Health gains

The two general approaches to improving health are the 'population' approach, focusing on measures to improve health through the community, and the 'high risk' approach, focusing on vulnerable individuals who are at a high risk of the condition or hazard. We promote a population approach for promoting the taking of folic acid before conception, and stopping smoking. We target vulnerable groups of individuals, such as looked-after children and those who have left care, to promote safe sex.[42]

The two approaches are not mutually exclusive and often need to be combined with legislation and community action. Health goals include:

- a good quality of life
- avoiding premature death
- equal opportunities for health.

Modifiable risk factors with potential health gains for pregnant women to reduce the risks of adverse effects on their foetus, as well as to enhance their own health, include:

- obesity
- lack of exercise
- excessive alcohol intake
- smoking.

Confidentiality

Confidentiality is a component of clinical governance that may be overlooked. Experienced health professionals and managers may assume that junior or new staff know all about confidentiality, but, of course, they may not. There are many tricky situations where one person asks for information about another's clinical condition – test results or a progress report – where it is not clear-cut as to whether this information should be supplied or withheld, or even if the person asked should acknowledge that the person enquired about is under their care. If the person in question is terminally ill and within a few days of death, the health professional will want to prepare the relatives; if the person with the terminal illness is functioning well, then their medical attendants will not be able to share medical information without the patient's express permission.

The Caldicott Committee Report[52] describes principles of good practice to safeguard confidentiality when information is being used for non-clinical purposes:

- justify the purpose
- do not use patient-identifiable information unless it is absolutely necessary
- use the minimum necessary patient-identifiable information
- access to patient-identifiable information should be on a strict need-to-know basis
- everyone with access to patient-identifiable information should be aware of his or her responsibilities.

Evidence-based culture: policy and practice

The key features of whether or not local guidelines worked in one initiative were that:[53]

- there was multidisciplinary involvement in drawing them up
- a well-described systematic review of the literature underpinned the guidelines with graded recommendations for best practice linked to the evidence
- ownership was nurtured at a national and local level
- a local implementation plan ensured that all the practicalities (time, staff, education and training, resources) were foreseen and met, stakeholders were supported, predictors of sustainability addressed – guideline usability, individualising guidelines to practitioners and patients.

Clinicians may rebel against new policies that they perceive as being out of line with patients' needs, and policy makers may become frustrated at the intransigence of those in practice – if there is a gulf between those driving policy and those responsible for practice. The evidence base justifying health policy and management decisions in relation to a particular service is just as important as the evidence base for the clinical care component of the service or the education of staff providing that service.

> Incorporating research-based evidence into everyday practice should promote policies on effective working and improve quality and a clinical governance culture.

- Be sure of the evidence for a proposed policy and the best way to implement it. Search for the evidence or set up a formal evaluation where there is insufficient evidence for the best way.
- Consult widely and early when any policy decision is being made, demonstrating how the input to that consultation was incorporated into the final policy.
- Base management and policy decisions on accurate information.
- Negotiate necessary changes in the organisation and management of the practice and carefully cascade information about the changes throughout the practice team or organisation.
- Provide adequate resources to underpin strategies to change practice, such as people to promote that change who have the right levels of knowledge and skills.
- Incorporate monitoring and evaluation of the change from the planning stage and throughout the activity.
- Find ways to maintain and reinforce the new practices, e.g. reminder systems, educational outreach programmes.
- Disseminate information about the change in ways that are appropriate to the nature and setting of the participants.

Accountability and performance

Health professionals – particularly GPs, pharmacists and dentists with their self-employed status – do not always realise that they are accountable to others from outside their own profession. But in fact they are accountable to:

- the general public – who are entitled to expect high standards of healthcare
- the profession – to maintain standards of knowledge and skills of the profession as a whole
- the government and employers – who expect high standards of healthcare from the workforce.

Midwives who believe that they are not accountable to others may be reluctant to collect the evidence to demonstrate that they are fit to practise, and that their working environment is fit to practise from, the basis of the evidence for revalidation of their professional qualifications. In addition, they may not co-operate with central NHS standards such as those set out in the National Service Frameworks or in *Standards for Better Health*.[54]

Identify and rectify underperformance at an early stage by:[55]

- regular appraisals (at least annually) linked into clinical governance and personal development plans. Appraisal is a process of regular meetings between manager and staff member with support for the benefit of the member of staff
- detecting those who have significant health problems and referring them for help
- systematic audit that detects individuals' performance as opposed to the overall performance of the practice or unit's team
- an open learning culture where team members are discouraged from covering up colleagues' inadequacies so that problems can be resolved at an early stage.

Health promotion

People may underestimate relative risks as applied to themselves and their own behaviour, e.g. many smokers accept the relationship between smoking tobacco and disease, but do not believe that they are personally at risk. People usually have a reasonable idea of the relative risks of various activities and behaviours, although their personal estimates of the magnitude of risks tend to be biased – small probabilities are often overestimated and high probabilities are often underestimated.[56]

> You need to understand the terms used to be able to extrapolate the messages from a research paper to explain the risks and benefits to others. You need critical appraisal skills to be able to form an opinion as to whether you can depend on the results from a research study. There are some publications where much of the work of interpreting results from research studies has been done for you in a reliable way (see www.ebandolier.com).[57]

Audit and evaluation

We should be looking for ways of assessing qualities like clinicians' and NHS managers' kindness, empathy, (clinical) reasoning and listening skills, as well as more tangible measures of the quality of care.

Analysis of critical incidents should focus on organisational factors as well as the performance of particular individuals.

Undertake regular audits of aspects of the structure, process and outcome of a service or development in your practice or department. See if you have achieved what you expected when you established the criteria and standards of the audit programme. Check out that you have completed the full cycle of the audit, including making changes and re-auditing.[58]

'When pathways and protocols are developed, an audit tool needs to be created to allow prospective evaluation of the care delivered and the outcomes achieved, including quality-of-life measures. Clinical teams and patients should be involved in determining how best to record outcomes, so that the measures developed address what really matters to patients.'[59]

Evaluation is essential to find out how well things are going. That could be checking out your experience in your post – such as the development of your knowledge and skills or how the team members work together, or how well you are delivering a service to patients. How else will you know if your efforts have been worthwhile, or if you could improve the way you do things? Incorporate evaluation into any plan to establish new staff posts, or where you vary what work staff do, right from the beginning. Keep your evaluation as simple as possible and avoid wasting resources on an unnecessarily bureaucratic type of evaluation.

Like all quality assurance processes, an evaluation should be:

- efficient, effective and economical – in relation to the costs and effectiveness of what you are evaluating as well as the evaluation process itself
- valid – evaluating what it is intended to measure
- reliable – producing consistent and accurate findings
- flexible and practical
- fair – not favouring any aspect; being inclusive
- in proportion – to the specific issues being evaluated
- accountable –specify lines of responsibility
- co-ordinated – with other development or review processes.[58]

Core requirements

You cannot deliver clinical governance without well-trained and competent staff, the right skill-mix of staff and a safe and comfortable working environment, all providing cost-effective care.

Following published referral guidelines may increase healthcare costs, which should be justifiable as cost-effective care when all direct and indirect costs are taken into account.

Your healthcare team can do much under the umbrella of clinical govern-ance to respond to the national challenges to improve:

- partnership: working together across the NHS to ensure the best possible care
- performance: acting to review and deliver higher standards of healthcare
- the professions and wider workforce: breaking down barriers between different disciplines
- patient care: access, convenient services, empowerment to take a full part in decision making about their own medical care and in planning and providing health services in general
- prevention: promoting healthy living across all sections of society and tackling variations in care.

Risk management

Risk management in general practice or a trust mainly centres on 'facts' rather than 'values' or 'preferences'. These are the facts about what the probability is that a hazard will give rise to harm – how bad is the risk, how likely is the risk, when will the risk happen, if ever, and how certain are we of our estimates about the risk? This applies just as much whether the risk is an environmental or organisational risk in the practice, or a clinical risk.[60]

Communicating and managing risks with individual patients is very much about finding ways to explain risks and elicit people's values and preferences, so that all these dimensions can be incorporated into the decisions they make themselves to take risks or choose between alternatives that involve different risks and benefits.[61] A well-functioning system through which patients can make complaints and receive feedback on the outcome should allow the practice or unit to reduce the risk of a recurrence.

2 How evidence-based care, clinical effectiveness and other components of clinical governance fit together: the primary care organisation's or trust's perspective[42]

The 14 components of clinical governance described apply just as much to the approach required by a trust as they do to practices and individual health professionals. But they must also set up:

- clear lines of responsibility and accountability for the overall quality of clinical care across their organisation for the area covered by their patient population
- a systematic approach to monitoring and developing clinical standards in practices
- a comprehensive programme of quality improvement systems including workforce planning and development
- education and training plans
- clear policies aimed at managing risk
- integrated procedures for all professional groups to identify and remedy poor performance
- a culture where education, research and sharing good practice are valued.

Clinical governance will be part of a culture of learning and the organisation will have an ethos of participation – for staff and patients to engage in quality improvement.

The Healthcare Commission and its predecessors work with trusts in England (with some duties in Wales) to improve quality through monitoring and service development. It covers primary care trusts (PCTs), hospital and specialist trusts, ambulance trusts, mental health trusts, care trusts and learning disability trusts. It does not include non-NHS organisations. The aim is to make sure that NHS trusts reach basic standards of healthcare and to encourage them to do better in future.

The annual health check is the Healthcare Commission's way of finding out how well NHS trusts are performing.[62] It checks how far they are meeting the Government's *Standards for Better Health*.[54]

Trusts receive a score of excellent, good, fair or weak for their standards of quality and use of resources, replacing the previous system of awarding a single 'star rating' to trusts. The quality element is derived from all of the components of the annual health check, except for use of resources. The quality of services is reviewed from a clinical point of view looking at how patients and the public actually experience them. The quality of care score covers core standards, existing targets, new national targets and the outcomes of improvement reviews and acute hospital portfolio studies. The use of resources element is based on an assessment of how effectively an organisation manages its financial resources.

The four high level questions at the core of the annual health check are:

- is care safe and clinically effective?
- are services accessible and patient focused?
- is public money used efficiently and effectively?
- is action being taken to improve and protect the health of local people and tackle inequalities?

To demonstrate good clinical governance, the primary care organisation or trust should be able to show that:

- users and carers believe that they are well cared for
- all staff feel included, listened to, and empowered in their roles
- all staff understand and own clinical governance
- there is an integrated strategy for the implementation of clinical governance
- the board has patient safety and service quality at the top of its agenda
- they identify and act on the areas of most concern to the organisation
- there is clear evidence of significant improvement in organisational performance.[63]

Practising midwives in England are subject to high-quality professional supervision through local supervising authorities (LSAs), which also provide an extra safety net and support for midwives themselves. The 13 regional LSAs are each hosted by one of the ten strategic health authorities (SHAs). The LSAs have a statutory duty to ensure the safety of midwifery practice towards women and children, and that midwives have up to date knowledge and skills. Their remit spans all practising midwives and not just those employed in the NHS. Each LSA has a local supervisory midwifery officer (LSAMO) who is professionally accountable to the Nursing and Midwifery Council (NMC), as well as being responsible to the chief executive of the host SHA. The LSAMO's role is about developing and sustaining effective clinical governance in respect of midwifery practice across their patch.

Threats to a coherent clinical governance programme in your practice or trust are:

- lack of consensus and teamwork in unit or practice
- lack of understanding of priorities and patients' needs
- staff thinking 'what's the point' if no resources for change?
- 'blame' culture – way of thinking
- geographic isolation of some staff and practices
- lack of trust and information about skills between health professions, or people's doubts about substitution involved in skill-mix
- suspicion of small practices or units that they will be criticised or have their priorities swamped by larger practices or the trust
- fear of new things/deficit in skills to cope with rapid change
- lack of time to fit new things in and get involved
- less well performing practices or units may find providing comparative data threatening
- clinical governance leads in primary care organisation or trust may be seen as 'know it alls' and 'do it alls' by others, who then leave them to it
- practitioners being unsure how best to proceed to blend clinical governance in with continuing professional development
- lack of ownership of the importance of clinical governance by 'ordinary' practitioners
- clinical governance being seen as a threat and as a top-down imposition by some
- lack of multidisciplinary culture or ownership – not all members of the practice or workplace team see themselves with a part to play in clinical governance
- anxieties about how information on performance will be used and interpreted
- staff sickness levels may create variations in the delivery of services and blips of underperformance if there is no backfill
- lack of systematic staff training with good strategic leadership
- patient expectations may exceed the capacity to deliver
- staff turnover may be detrimental, e.g. loss of experience in applying disease registers and recall systems
- some small isolated practices or specialty units may find it hard to share information and resources with peers
- lack of opportunities/willingness to learn about clinical governance in some practices or units
- low level of patient or public involvement in practice or unit, so standards are set by healthcare staff rather than the public
- worries about identifying weaknesses within team or to employer or outside person which may become source of blame

- health professionals may not see the wider context of the contributions of non-health organisations to improving health, nor understand each others' roles or the potential of the services each offers.

A National Audit Office report[64] found that there were clear indications of changes to a culture supporting clinical governance and that individual components of clinical governance were mainly in place in most trusts. The range of achievements included:

- clinical quality issues being more mainstream
- structures and organisational arrangements to make clinical governance happen being in place
- clinical governance being well established and embedded in the corporate systems of virtually all trusts
- progress in the development of a more co-ordinated, coherent and consistent clinical governance strategy in trusts.

One hospital approach to clinical governance was to reform the senior committee structure to reflect:[65]

- leadership at different levels
- multidisciplinary style
- active co-ordination of the different elements of the committee, and of the hospital
- sharing of work across the service.

To achieve this, lead roles and responsibilities were allotted so that:

- evidence-based practice was led by a consultant psychiatrist
- risk management was led by a forensic psychologist
- a nurse manager led on policy and procedure
- the senior occupational therapist led on clinical audit
- a general manager led on user issues and complaints.

The Healthcare Concordat is a voluntary agreement between organisations that regulate, audit, inspect or review elements of health and healthcare in England. So, inspections are co-ordinated with other reviews and collections of data and focus on the experiences of patients, other users of services and carers. Inspections support improvements in quality and performance, and are targeted and proportionate. The website includes a range of tools, including a scheduling tool which allows signatory bodies to co-ordinate their visits to providers of healthcare.[66]

Full signatories to the Healthcare Concordat are the:

- Healthcare Commission
- Audit Commission
- National Audit Office
- Mental Health Act Commission
- Commission for Social Care Inspection
- Health and Safety Executive
- NHS Litigation Authority
- Academy of Medical Royal Colleges
- Post Graduate Medical Education and Training Board
- Conference of Postgraduate Deans
- General Medical Council
- Human Fertilisation and Embryology Authority
- NHS Counter Fraud and Security Management Service
- Skills for Health.

3 Research Governance Framework for Health and Social Care

Research is essential to health and wellbeing and to the development of modern and effective services. Just as clinical governance aims to continually improve the standards of clinical care and to reduce unacceptable variations in clinical practice, *research governance* aims to continually improve the standards of research and to reduce unacceptable variations in research practice. Research governance applies across health and social care and aims to enhance the partnership between health services and science.

The *Research Governance Framework for Health and Social Care*[67] defines the broad principles of good research governance and is the key to ensuring that health and social care research is conducted to high scientific and ethical standards. The Research Governance Framework spans the responsibilities of individuals and organisations involved in research, outlines delivery systems and standards to improve research quality and safeguard the public and describes local and national monitoring systems. It involves enhancing ethical and scientific quality, promoting good practice, reducing adverse incidents, ensuring lessons are learned and preventing poor performance and misconduct. The *Research Governance Framework for Health and Social Care* is summarised in the box below.

Research Governance Framework for Health and Social Care

What does research governance do?

- sets standards in research and defines the mechanisms to deliver those standards
- describes the monitoring and assessment arrangements
- improves research quality and safeguards the public by:
  - enhancing the ethical and scientific quality of research
  - promoting good practice in research
  - reducing adverse incidents in research and ensuring lessons are learned
  - preventing poor performance and misconduct in research.

Who is research governance for?

- managers and staff, in all professional groups, no matter how senior or junior and for all those who:
  - participate in research
  - host research in their organisation
  - fund research proposals or infrastructure
  - manage research
  - undertake research
- everyone working in all health and social care research environments, including:
  - primary care
  - secondary care
  - tertiary care
  - social care
  - public health.

What does research governance cover?

- ethics
- science
- information
- health, safety and employment
- finance and intellectual property.

Where can I get research governance documents?

- An updated edition of the *Research Governance Framework for Health and Social Care* for **England** is on the web at: www.dh.gov.uk
- The Scottish Executive *Research Governance Framework for Health and Community Care* is on the web at: www.show.scot.nhs.uk/CSO/Publications/ResGov/Framework/RGFEdTwo.pdf
- The *Research Governance Framework for Health and Social Care* in **Wales** is being updated and may be accessed through www.dh.gov.uk
- The *Research Governance Framework for Health and Social Care* in **Northern Ireland** is at: www.centralserviceagency.n-i.nhs.uk/files/rdo_whats_new/file/RGF_061106.pdf

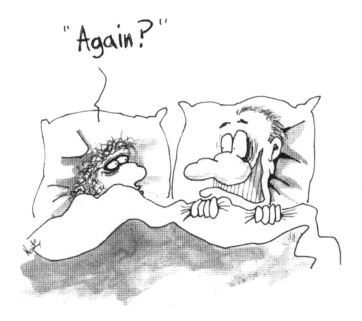

Once you've tried to apply clinical effectiveness – you'll want to do it again!

Stage 7

Focusing on your revalidation – where clinical governance fits

Times are a-changing with the expectation that midwives will be required to undergo revalidation of their professional status to ensure their continuing fitness to practise in the near future. The Nursing and Midwifery Council's current process of re-registration every three years with the post-registration education and practice (PREP) standards requirement for a minimum number of 35 hours spent on continuing professional development (CPD) in the three years prior to renewal of professional registration, will change to a more exacting system whereby midwives, nurses and others provide evidence that they have kept up to date with clinical and professional developments and are fit to practise.

The primary purpose of professional regulation of midwives and other health professionals is to ensure patient safety. Regulation is the set of systems and activities intended to ensure that healthcare practitioners have the necessary knowledge, skills, attitudes and behaviours to provide healthcare safely. The core activities of regulation are:

- keeping the register of members admitted to practice
- determining standards of education and training for admission to practice
- giving advice about standards of conduct and performance
- administering procedures (including making rules) relating to misconduct, unfitness to practice and similar matters.[68]

Revalidation is the process by which a regulated professional periodically has to demonstrate that they remain fit to practise – in terms of competence and performance, health and conduct/character.[69] The three main purposes are to:

1 ensure that individual health professionals provide minimally acceptable standards of care in terms of the safety and quality of care given
2 reassure patients and the public that health professionals deserve their trust; sustain their confidence by the demonstrable impartiality of the regulatory system

3 improve the quality of patient care through striving for best practice by: sustaining improvements in performance via measurement and feedback and by identifying and addressing poor practice or bad behaviour.[68,69]

A review of the regulation of non-medical professionals in the UK envisages a framework that spans CPD, appraisal, and revalidation too. Their revalidation system is expected to start after that of doctors has been introduced – so, after 2010. The recommendations were about:

- regulation of the professions across one integrated framework
- more independent adjudication regarding fitness to practise cases
- standardising the content and enhancing the value of workplace appraisal
- revalidation for every registered health professional, including midwives.[68,69]

New roles in the NHS such as maternity assistants urgently need statutory regulation. NHS employers will need to put in place systems to monitor non-medical professional staff for their revalidation. It is expected that evidence to support the revalidation of midwives will be incorporated within normal staff management and clinical governance systems, with their employers providing recommendations as to their continuing fitness to practise, to their professional regulator. Regulatory bodies will develop direct revalidation arrangements for any health professionals who practise in a private capacity; and NHS primary care organisations will oversee revalidation processes for self-employed professionals who contract with them to provide services such as dentists and optometrists.[69]

How the revalidation process for midwives is set up and runs will reflect the nature and level of risks to patient safety from their scope of practice (see Table 5). The Department of Health will discuss with each profession and its regulator (that is, the NMC for midwives) the arrangements for their revalidation. Appraisal will be a key component, and in England, the Knowledge and Skills Framework (KSF) will be central to the framework of evidence of competence. The Council for Healthcare Regulatory Excellence (CHRE) will work with the regulators, the professions and all four countries of the UK. A UK revalidation steering group will be set up to develop and co-ordinate this work.

The KSF is a generic framework that focuses on how you apply your knowledge and skills in your post as a midwife. Your annual development review should already include appraisal, assessment against the KSF and production of a personal development plan (PDP) using the KSF as a developmental tool. So the information and evidence that you collect over the year under the various components of the KSF relevant to your job role, should be the basis of your future revalidation.[70]

Table 5   Risk factors that trusts and primary care organisations may consider in deciding the intensiveness of revalidation for particular staff.[68]

Higher risk	Lower risk
High level of responsibility for patient safety inherent in scope of practice	Low level of responsibility for patient safety inherent in scope of practice
Leaders of clinical teams	Team members
Practitioners who practise outside managed environments such as a hospital or clinic	Practitioners who practise within such environments
Practitioners whose work environment is not subject to NHS standards of clinical governance	Practitioners whose work environment is subject to NHS standards of clinical governance
Practitioners who are frequently alone with patients (including in their homes)	Practitioners who always work in a team or do not work face to face with patients
Unsupervised practitioners/posts	Supervised practitioners/posts
Practitioners in their first few years of registration (and possibly also their last few, according to some)	Registrants in mid (or late?) career
Recent adverse findings by NMC	Clean regulatory record
Recent appraisal or performance review shows concern about performance	Good performance record
Practitioners using invasive, high-risk interventions	Practitioners using low-risk interventions

Moving from appraisal to revalidation

The major purpose of appraisal is to identify the professional development and learning needs of a midwife and to ensure these are acted upon. Box 2 describes the main features of appraisal which should contribute to ensuring that:

- midwives' practice is safe
- midwives' practice is of a good standard
- opportunities to improve practice /performance are taken.

Box 2   Features of appraisal.[70]

The different features of appraisal can be broadly mapped across to the following improvement processes:

- professional development
- clinical governance
- performance management
- assessment and assurance of minimum standards
- informal and formal developmental relationships.

Following the White Paper,[69] the appraisal process is expected to be developed so that it contains both summative and formative assessments. With the summative component, a midwife would include assessments that show that their performance has met specific standards. With the formative component, they would look forward to plan and carry out any changes that might need to be made according to what the formative assessment revealed.

Good practice in appraisal*

Good practice in relation to the appraisal process is when there is an organisational commitment to a quality assured appraisal system that is part of the clinical governance framework. Then there will be consistent good practice in relation to:

- training of appraisers
- handling of concerns about fitness to practise arising during an appraisal
- internal quality assurance, in particular in reporting to the board of a NHS employer or contractor
- external quality assurance
- effective administrative and IT support to the overall process.

To be effective the appraisal process must be challenging.[71]

The outcome of an appraisal must be a personal development plan that outlines what the individual should do to make the improvements that have been identified as necessary. This places an onus on both the individual doctor and the employing/contracting body to take action. An important part of the appraisal process is a review of the previous PDP to ensure that all requisite actions have been taken since the last appraisal.

Important areas to cover in appraisal include actions to:

- maintain your skills and your level of service to patients
- develop or acquire new skills
- change or improve your existing practice
- address all areas of particular importance to the nature of your work.

The success of any clinical service is mainly determined by the performance of its human resource – the people working in the department or practice or elsewhere in the NHS. The trust/PCO, and NHS in general, needs information about its staff concerning their performance in the job, their future potential,

---

* Much of the section that follows is from the working papers of Mason A, Chambers R, Conlon M, Borgardts I. *Principles underlying the standards to be used in appraisal*, a series of papers commissioned by The Academy of Medical Royal Colleges of the Career Grade Doctor Appraisal Forum. www.appraisalsupport.nhs.uk included with their kind permission.

and their education, training and development needs. Midwives need to know what is expected of them, how they are perceived to have performed, how they are valued as members of the team and whether there is anything they could do to improve their performance or to develop their careers.

In terms of evidence used in appraisal, good practice is using information about:

- an individual midwife's workload, such as use of drugs and outcomes of care
- standards of record keeping
- reflective practice – outline description of focus, scope, application
- involvement of an individual midwife in local or national systems of quality improvement and safety assurance

and multi-source (360°) feedback from:

- patients
- those being taught, trained, appraised or assessed
- colleagues concerning patient care
- colleagues concerning management responsibilities.

If information about clinical activity is to be used in appraisal it must relate to:

- the quality and safety of the care delivered
- activities for which a specific midwife is responsible, which can be accurately attributed to that individual
- the aims of the appraisal process.

Where clinical governance fits with revalidation

Appraisal is a key part of a local clinical governance framework. Having an effective quality assured appraisal system for midwives shows an organisation's commitment to excellence and provides a mechanism to:

- assist midwives to identify improvements that they need to make in their everyday work and their own specialty
- ensure that requisite action is taken to make the improvements.

The aims of both midwives and managers with respect to the provision of clinical services, from both individual and organisational perspectives, should include:

- continuous quality improvement
- assurance of safety

- reduction of risk
- minimisation of costs (without detriment to the other objectives).

If clinical services are to meet these aims, they should:

- use effective evidence-based interventions
- be delivered by clinically and managerially competent health professionals focused on their patients' welfare
- be planned around patient-centred clinical pathways
- be enabled by efficient operational systems supporting the pathways.

Clinical governance is carried out through a framework which ensures that NHS bodies are accountable for continuously improving the quality of their services and safeguarding their standards of care.

Effective clinical governance requires information about the care provided, in terms of:

- patient experience
- clinical outcomes
- operational efficiency.

Then armed with this information, requiring clinicians and clinical teams to:

- assess the quality of care they provide
- reflect on this experience and learn from successes and failures
- apply the lessons learned to improve the quality of services provided.[45]

Key elements of a clinical governance ethos in any NHS setting include:

- the creation of a culture or environment throughout an organisation in which excellence will flourish
- effective leadership at all levels and effective multidisciplinary team working of an organisation – a hospital, primary care organisation or practice, etc.
- uniformly good participation in clinical audit by all clinicians and managers
- provision of information about the care provided and health professionals providing it so that the need for improvement can be identified
- meaningful engagement of patients using the service
- proactive risk assessment and management of clinical processes and the environment in which care is delivered
- identification of actions that need to be taken to ensure improvements are made
- setting up of mechanisms to ensure requisite actions are taken.[45,71]

Clinical governance issues that will be highlighted in the context of re-validation include:

- supporting those who want to register complaints or concerns; investigating these complaints and concerns
- helping individual midwives to remedy their shortcomings where possible
- making more systematic use of clinical outcomes data relating to individual teams or practitioners
- ensuring information about a midwife's performance is brought together and where appropriate and subject to strict safeguards, shared between healthcare organisations and with the director lead for midwives or equivalent
- separating the investigation of potential poor performance or misconduct from formal decision-making processes, to protect patients.[69]

There is a national push for patient safety. The National Patient Safety Agency (NPSA), and 28 other Royal Colleges, faculties and health organisations have signed up to improve the safety of healthcare in the UK. They pledge to 'minimise the risk of harm to patients occurring as a consequence of health-care, and aspire to create one of the "safest health services in the world".' This includes incorporating patient safety into training and education programmes, and encouraging the open reporting of incidents without any recrimination. Key elements of development include:

- ensuring appropriate treatments are offered with as near to possible 100% reliability
- minimising the risk of errors leading to avoidable adverse effects of treatment or investigation
- promoting a culture of incident reporting and patient safety
- ensuring a more consistent response to failures of systems and major systems weaknesses in the NHS.[72,73]

Continuing professional development (CPD)

CPD is 'concerned with the acquisition, enhancement and maintenance of knowledge, skills and attitudes by professional practitioners'; its broad aims are to enhance professionals' performance and optimise the outcomes of their practice[74] as you saw in Stage 6. It will be increasingly important that you can demonstrate the quality of your CPD and how you apply it in your everyday work for revalidation purposes. You should be able to show that the learning you have undertaken was of the right quality, scope and level to address gaps in your knowledge, skills and service needs. And furthermore, you should keep evidence that you did in fact learn and apply your updated knowledge and skills appropriately to improve the quality of care you provide in your personal professional portfolio.

Differentiating appraisal and assessment

Assessment and appraisal are two distinct processes with different aims. Assessment measures progress based on relevant curricula, while appraisal focuses on the person and their professional needs. 'Appraisal is ... an ongoing, two-way process involving reflection on an individual's performance, identification of education needs and planning for personal development. Appraisal allows midwives to take time to reflect on their performance and skills and examine how successes in particular areas can be transferred to other areas of their work. Assessment involves the measurement of an individual's performance at a particular point in time, usually against predetermined standards. Different types of assessment measure different aspects of being a midwife. Results of assessments can feed into appraisals if appropriate.'[75]

With revalidation, the purpose of the assessment is to determine if the midwife is fit to practise; and the evidence will be partly drawn from the summative assessment aspects that will feature in appraisal. Table 6 compares the purpose and other characteristics of appraisal and assessment; whilst Table 7 captures some of the key differences in features and approach between assessment and appraisal.

Work-based assessment encompasses what you really do/how you perform (e.g. multi-source feedback) as well as what you show you can do/your competence.

Preparing for appraisal and revalidation[70]

The secret to preparing well is to collect evidence about the standards of your practice throughout the year, so that you do yourself justice across the whole range of your work. There should be an opportunity for you and your appraiser to exchange information and documents before the appraisal.

Your appraiser should be able to understand the pressures of your work created by the demands of providing patient care with limited resources and other factors that are beyond your control. Collect facts about any such pressures or resource problems, rather than impressions. Be specific rather than whinge. Then your evidence about the nature of the barriers that hinder you and other colleagues from achieving best practice can be taken into

Table 6 Characteristics of appraisal and assessment.[75]

Feature	Appraisal	Assessment
Prime purpose	Developmental 'Informing progress'	Judging achievement 'Summing up'
Participants	Appraiser and appraisee	Learner and third party
Methods used	Structured conversation	Varied
Areas covered	Educational, personal and professional development, career progress, employment (appraisee's agenda)	Learning objectives (third party agenda)
Process informed by	Appraisee's self-assessment, day to day observation by others, other work related inputs, results of assessments and examinations	Outcome of standard objective tests
Standards of achievement	Internal (personal to appraisee) and negotiated with appraiser	Pre-determined by assessing body
Output of the process	Record of appraisal having taken place, agreed PDP	Pass/fail
Confidential to learner?	Yes, in the main	No
Review/appeal	No need, as decisions should be joint ones	Yes
Outcome	Enhanced educational, personal and professional development	Proceed to next stage

account. That evidence from appraisals should also be collated across your trust to inform its business planning and workforce and educational strategies.

Record your personal and professional development throughout the year under the same headings required for your appraisal to avoid unnecessary work in preparing for appraisal and revalidation. Collect facts rather than unsubstantiated opinions, so that the appraisal exercise is fair. Obtain them from a broad base of sources or informants to counter any criticism of selective reporting. Appraisal and job planning should fit together with the outcomes of each informing the other.

Putting the data together

Present the evidence for your appraisal and revalidation as a portfolio of your activity for the year. This is an important document and needs time and

Table 7 Assessment versus appraisal of an individual.[75]

Factors	Assessment	Appraisal
Valid	√	?
Reliable	√	?
Practicable	√	√
Fair	√	?
Useful	√	√
Acceptable	√	√
Appropriate	√	?
Judgemental	√	?
Formative	Not usually; but can be	√
Timing	As required	Regular
Scope	Specific	Wide, comprehensive
Methodology	Varied	Generic
Relationship with other reviews	May relate or stand alone	Inter-relates
Include review of behaviour	Not necessarily	Must
Learning opportunity	Yes – strengths and weaknesses	Yes – self-assessment and peer's view of extent of achievements

? = depends on quality of appraiser; and requirements of employing organisation

consideration spent in its construction. Avoid trying to gather all the information in the few weeks immediately preceding your appraisal interview. Look for any updates on the websites of the Royal College of Midwifery or other professional organisations. You will probably find that over time in the run up to the launch of revalidation in say 2010–11, the requirements become more specific as to what is essential evidence from a personal practice perspective, what is essential from an organisational view and what is optional. The NHS Clinical Governance Support Team has done a lot of preparatory work on this for doctors and it is worth looking at its website for other ideas too: www. appraisalsupport.nhs.uk

For instance, when thinking about proving your good clinical care, you might include:

- essential evidence (personal): a clinical audit that demonstrates your personal performance for good clinical care matched against professional guidance or NICE guidelines as featured in your PDP. Include a reflective piece as to standards reached and how you will improve your practice as appropriate. This might be a full audit cycle

- essential evidence (organisational): a key organisational audit generated by your trust/primary care organisation/practice with reflection on how your own performance compared with that of others and your thoughts on the strengths and weaknesses of the service described by the data; and plan to make changes, then review those changes. It may be that the organisational audit is one specified by your employing/host organisation
- optional evidence: other personal audits or significant event audits (from personal or organisational perspectives) with your reflections on the findings and your subsequent action plans; and review changes made.

A successful portfolio needs to have a definite and logical structure and include a content page and sections for easy reference. Midwives may be able to organize their own portfolio or employing trusts may define a structure.

Necessary preparation

One of the problems of preparing for appraisal and revalidation is the wealth of information and evidence required, and your lack of time to collect and compile it. Initially it requires organisation; decide what you need to collect, what you can collect, then how you are going to collect it. Try to establish systems of data collection that can be repeated each year. Liaise closely with your trust as they may already have the data that you require or may already have defined data that they require should be collected to illustrate your activity.

Figure 3 gives an outline of how to prepare for your appraisal as a hospital clinician. Adapt the top boxes of the middle column if you are working in other settings.

The data you collect should aim to reflect all aspects of your practice. The nature of the data will depend on what resources the trust will provide and what data can be reasonably collected individually without you committing a large amount of time and personal effort. The data then needs to be mapped against the domains required for your appraisal. One piece of evidence of your performance at work may map to several of the domains.

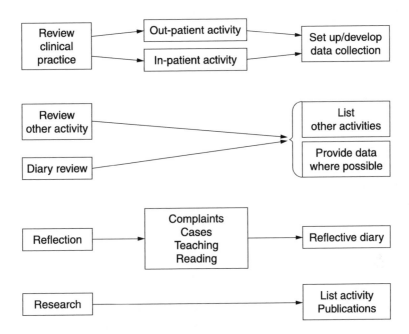

Figure 3:   Preparing for the appraisal process as a hospital clinician.

Compiling an effective personal development plan (PDP)[44,70]

A PDP is an essential part of your appraisal and revalidation documentation. Having made a lot of effort to present your data and review your achievements and current practice, you will want to draw up a PDP for the next 12 months, endorsed by your appraiser. The scope of the plan will probably be set by your trust and professional requirements but you should not sign-up to it until you are comfortable with the content – and its formative and developmental nature.

Both the start and end points for appraisal should be the PDP. Part of the appraisal is the review of progress based on the previous PDP and this is a useful method of getting what resources and support you need out of your employing or host organisation. Headings for a PDP should include as a minimum:

* review of progress and previously agreed objectives since last appraisal
* objectives: short-term, long-term
* resources required
* timetabled action plan.

The close of the appraisal should include a definitive statement in your PDP as to what you should achieve in the next 12 months and the agreement of both you and your appraiser as to how this will be achieved. If you are employed, it is important to hold the trust or your employer to this agreement.

If you have kept on top of your personal development plan over the last year, you will already have justified what you plan to learn as a priority in the next 12 months. Allow some space in your plan to become updated on changes in regulations or in relation to additional responsibilities you could not have predicted at your last appraisal. So, there should be few changes, unless your own personal priorities are not synchronised with those of your primary care organisation, hospital trust, or employer.

Use triangulation to strengthen the evidence of your performance. If you have at least three pieces of evidence pointing in a particular direction that will increase the accuracy.

To decide what you can collect requires that you review all aspects of your clinical practice. If you supply the appraiser before or at the interview with two box files and a carrier bag of papers and expect the appraiser to sort through it for evidence of your good practice – think again! You have just demonstrated your unfamiliarity with the appraisal and revalidation processes and that you are lacking in organisational skills. You will be unable to demonstrate your good practice if the appraiser cannot identify it easily.

How to identify your development and service needs

Self-assessment using a rating scale

Self-assessment can be criticised as inaccurate or biased. But it is useful for establishing areas of your work where you do not feel confident. You might draw up a list of skills that are relevant to your job, or use a skills summary that has already been developed for use in training situations. Many trainees are assessed in this way when first starting a job so that they and their trainers can draw up an initial learning programme.

It is probably easier to self-assess your practical skills than those associated with clinical management, clinical judgement or professional values, etc. However, reflecting on all the parameters of your job might enable you to see some gaps, or to appreciate areas you had not previously considered as relevant. You can follow up your self-assessment with other checks by asking colleagues for their perspectives of your work (peer review or multi-source feedback) or gather more objective measures.

You might try to rate your knowledge and ability with specific clinical conditions. You will tend to consider common conditions, but if it is rare, it may be of even more importance that you manage it well. Your self-assessment of your management of a clinical condition might include:

- assessment of the patient and diagnosis
- providing or arranging investigations
- providing or arranging treatment
- emergency treatment
- where the limits of your competence lie and when you should refer
- what records you keep
- prevention of that condition.

Self-assess your level of confidence on the 1–5 scale shown by circling the appropriate number (1 = not at all confident ...... 5 = very confident)

Specific practical skills (examples only – revise or add yours)

I can identify mental illness during pregnancy	1....2....3....4....5
I can use a sphygmomanometer – according to best practice guidelines	1....2....3....4....5
I can perform a vaginal examination	1....2....3....4....5
I can undertake basic cardiopulmonary resuscitation	1....2....3....4....5
I can perform neonatal resuscitation	1....2....3....4....5
I can recognise and repair perineal trauma	1....2....3....4....5
I can set up a syntocinon regime correctly	1....2....3....4....5
I can safely administer drugs	1....2....3....4....5
Other (you add):	1....2....3....4....5

Patient management skills

I can share decision making with patients about their clinical management, as a matter of course	1....2....3....4....5
I can enable patient concordance, as a routine	1....2....3....4....5
I can signpost patients to reliable sources of information about their condition(s)	1....2....3....4....5
Other (you add):	1....2....3....4....5

Clinical judgement

I can undertake appropriate examination and investigations for a typical patient who consults me	1....2....3....4....5
I can assess whether a patient requires a high or low risk care pathway	1....2....3....4....5
I can respond appropriately to requests for urgent care	1....2....3....4....5
Other (you add):	1....2....3....4....5

Communication skills

I can complete, store and retain records	1....2....3....4....5
I can give health education	1....2....3....4....5
I can communicate effectively with patients	1....2....3....4....5
I can communicate effectively with colleagues in my workplace	1....2....3....4....5
I can develop effective professional working across boundaries	1....2....3....4....5
Other (you add):	1....2....3....4....5

Continued

Personal and professional growth

I can identify strengths/weaknesses in my performance .... 1....2....3....4....5
I can make an action plan to redress my weaknesses and complete it ... 1....2....3....4....5
I can develop my own knowledge and skills .... 1....2....3....4....5
I can contribute to evaluation, guidelines and procedures .... 1....2....3....4....5
I can understand and contribute to audit .... 1....2....3....4....5
Other (you add): .... 1....2....3....4....5

Organisational skills

I know my limitations and can refer appropriately .... 1....2....3....4....5
I can manage my time well .... 1....2....3....4....5
I can manage and prioritise demands .... 1....2....3....4....5
Other (you add): .... 1....2....3....4....5

Professional values

I can describe my ethical principles .... 1....2....3....4....5
I prioritise patient safety at all times .... 1....2....3....4....5
I can maintain confidentiality in relation to patient information .. 1....2....3....4....5
I maintain accountability in accordance with NMC rules and regulations ... 1....2....3....4....5
Other (you add): .... 1....2....3....4....5

What do other people think of your self-assessment of your skills?

What are your priorities for improving your skills?

Figure 4:   Self-assessment rating scale.

Multi-source feedback (also known as 360° feedback)[75]

There is a great deal of research about the validity of this methodology. Essentially it examines attitudes and behaviour of you as a midwife as perceived by those you work with (and maybe your patients too), as illustrated by the arrangement in Box 3.

Box 3   Illustrative example of participants in 360° feedback.

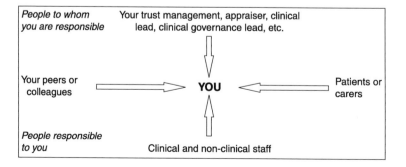

The wider the spread of people giving feedback, the more rounded the picture. Each individual gives a feedback questionnaire to a minimum number of people in each of the groups participating in the feedback exercise. An independent person then collects and collates the questionnaires and discusses the results with the individual. The main disadvantage of this method is that it can sometimes be spoilt by malicious comments against which individuals cannot readily defend themselves. The person facilitating the feedback should be trained to do so. Use the principles of good practice listed in Box 4 to determine which type of multi-source feedback questionnaire to use if you or your organisation have a choice.

Box 4   Principles for formative multi-source feedback (MSF) systems (e.g. for use within appraisal).[71]

The principles which apply to MSF being used formatively within regular appraisal where the data comes from professional colleagues include:

- the purpose of the MSF must be clear and widely understood
- MSF is just one part of the 'information for appraisal' system
- MSF works best in a supportive organisational culture
- the description of the 'domains' must be clear and appropriate
- the number of domains should be limited
- the scale points must be clear, appropriate and consistently construed
- allow free text comments
- psychometrical robustness of the system is a valuable attribute
- raters should be well-informed, well-chosen, representative and fair
- ratings should be confidential but not anonymous
- results of formative MSF must be presented by someone skilled and trained in feedback and should be compared with self-assessment
- the system should operate sufficiently frequently to have an impact
- the system should work well and continue to evolve.[11]

Analysis of your strengths, weaknesses, opportunities and threats (SWOT)[70,76]

You can undertake a SWOT analysis of your own performance or that of your team in your department, practice or trust. Brainstorm the strengths, weaknesses, opportunities and threats of the situation on your own, or with a workmate or mentor, or with a group of colleagues – enter what you come up with for each empty quadrant as in Table 8.

Your strengths and weaknesses will relate to your knowledge, experience and expertise in: decision making, communication, inter-professional relationships, political matters, timekeeping, organisational, teaching and research skills. In a positive moment, you might think of your weaknesses as being challenges.

Opportunities might relate to your unexploited potential strengths, expected changes, options for career development pathways, hobbies and interests that you might usefully expand.

Threats will include factors and circumstances that prevent you from achieving your aims for personal, professional and service development.

Prioritise the important factors. Draw up goals and a timed action plan to make the most of strengths and opportunities and combat weaknesses and threats.

A SWOT analysis might focus on your weaknesses in an area such as patient and public involvement. Your objective then might be to learn how to explain risks to patients or involve them more in decision making about their clinical management, for instance.

Table 8   SWOT analysis.

Strengths	Weaknesses
Opportunities	Threats

Significant event audit[77,78]

Significant event audit is a structured approach you can use to review events that have occurred that are relevant to your work. That way you can identify areas of your work that require improvement.

To carry out a significant event audit, meet up with others who are also involved to review that event. It is a learning exercise – to be done in an atmosphere of trust and respect and not to apportion blame. If the patient(s) or those caring for the patient(s) are identifiable (and they usually are) then all involved must agree that what is discussed is confidential and any report must be anonymised. Then discuss everything that happened following the steps in Figure 5:

- management of the event
- any opportunities for prevention
- follow-up
- implications for the patient, relatives and community
- actions of clinical and non-clinical members of the team
- action(s) that should be taken as a result of the review
- how action(s) (if required) will be evaluated or monitored.

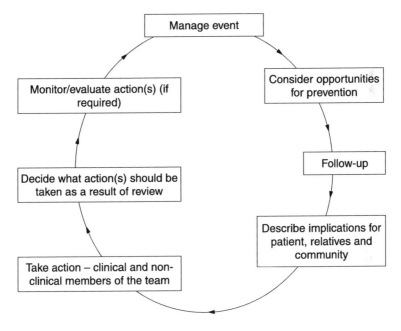

Figure 5:   Significant event audit cycle.

Some significant events are adverse incidents. These are events where something has clearly gone wrong, and you need to establish what happened, what was preventable and what changes are needed. Some adverse incidents may reveal only minor risks or ones that would occur extremely infrequently and will be judged by the team as not requiring any changes. But an adverse event that is very serious, however rare, will require action.

In hospital settings, a range of confidential reviews such as those relating to maternity events, deaths and suicides provide useful opportunities to review your roles in teamwork and other issues.

Risk management reporting of adverse events and near misses should be part of routine clinical governance management. In risk management reporting there should be an easily identifiable route for action that should include:

- identify and record the adverse incident or near miss
- report to an overall monitoring body in the workplace or organisation
- analysis of the incident
- group together any similar occurrences to determine any trends
- discuss any necessary changes with people involved
- implement any changes necessary.

Audit, e.g. of protocols and guidelines

Audit is about setting standards for your performance, finding out how you are doing, searching to find out best practice, making the changes and then re-auditing the care given to patients in the future with the same problem, as in Figure 6.[78]

The five steps of the audit cycle are to:

1 describe the criteria and standards you're trying to achieve
2 measure your current performance in providing care or services – in an objective way
3 compare your performance against criteria and standards
4 identify if there is a need for change – to performance, adjustment of criteria or standards, resources, available data
5 make any required changes as necessary and re-audit later.

Audit can be undertaken in a variety of ways – for example:

- case note analysis. This gives you insight into your current practice. It can be a retrospective review of a random selection of notes, or a prospective survey of consecutive patients with the same condition as they present
- criteria based audit. This compares clinical practice with specific standards, guidelines or protocols. Re-audit of changes should demonstrate improvements in the quality of patient care. You could compare the proportion of patients meeting your criteria for good care over intervals of time. Consult with all those involved – patients and carers, nurses, doctors, reception staff, therapists, pharmacists, etc. – to put plans into action, improve what you do and then re-audit.

You can use audit to review, evaluate and improve patient care in a systematic way, to improve their healthcare and quality of life. Performance is often broken down into the three aspects of structure, process and outcome for the purposes of audit. Structural audits might concern resources such as

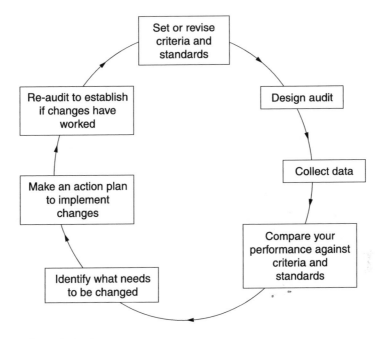

Figure 6:   The audit cycle.

equipment, premises, skills, people, etc. Process audits focus on what was done to the patient; for instance, clinical protocols and guidelines. Audits of outcomes consider the impact of care or services on the patient and might include patient satisfaction, health gains, effectiveness of care or services.[77,78]

The direction of clinical audit should be to promote:

- a clear patient focus
- greater multi-professional working
- an inter-sectoral approach across primary, secondary and continuing care boundaries
- close links with education and professional development
- integration of information about clinical effectiveness, cost effectiveness, variations in practice, outcome measurement and critical appraisal skills.

You might determine your learning needs (and those of other team members) by collecting examples of all the protocols or guidelines that exist somewhere in the workplace and rationalising them so that you have a common set. There are bound to be associated learning needs with taking this common approach to enable everyone to be aware of the documents, understand their roles and responsibilities for the various pathways in their everyday work, and be able to adhere to the protocols or guidelines, or justify any deviation.

Patient satisfaction surveys.

One person, such as the practice or ward manager, clerical assistant or secretary, should take charge of the organisation of regular patient satisfaction surveys. In order to ensure that information from different sites is comparable, and that the results of changes can be monitored before and after surveys, it is essential that the survey is undertaken in a standardised manner and that all staff involved know what to do.

It is preferable to use a questionnaire that has been tried and tested previously. Designing your own version risks including flawed and ambiguous questions that may give misleading results. The results from a tested questionnaire are more likely to be valid and reliable, and it will save you a lot of time. Results can be compared with those previously obtained and can be used to show change. Findings can also be compared with those obtained by other health professionals using the same questionnaire – so that you can compare your results with theirs. Some questionnaires already available are described below. You can use the results to discuss with colleagues in what ways you might need to alter your consultation style.

Some questionnaires are available to feedback on health professionals' performance and quality of their care and services.

- SHEFFPAT was initially developed for use in paediatrics, but has been used more widely in hospital and general practice. It is designed to measure the quality of the consultation. In a review of questionnaires designed to gather feedback from patients on individual doctors it was rated highly for its content, development and testing capacity.[79]
- The Patient Enablement Instrument (PEI) consists of a short questionnaire that was initially designed for use in primary care. The generic questions are designed to assess patients' ability to understand and cope with their illness. It can be used without permission; see Howie *et al.*[80] for details about how it should be administered and scored.
- The Patient Satisfaction Questionnaire (PSQ-18) includes items relating to patient satisfaction with doctors, as well as access, appointments, facilities and nurses, plus general satisfaction with the service as a whole.[81]
- The NHS Patient Survey Programme in England is run by local NHS trusts carrying out local surveys asking patients for their views on their recent experiences of the health service. The surveys are developed centrally for the Healthcare Commission; over a million people have taken part. So the results of local surveys can be compared across the country and over time (see www.nhssurveys.org).[79,82]
- Patient satisfaction questionnaires have been developed by some of the medical Royal Colleges as relevant to their specialties. Make sure that they have been validated.

- Some trusts have been using questionnaires developed by their audit departments. Many of these have not been subjected to testing or review and may not give valid or reliable results. Check before use! Some primary care organisations insist that practices use a particular questionnaire so that results across their area are comparable.

Check that the survey you select does focus on areas of practice that patients consider to be important. Recent research has confirmed that the public consider listening and good communication skills, providing a good standard of practice and care, and technical competence as fundamental to good practice.[82,83] So the questions in the survey you select should cover these areas.

You may want to find out yourself what tool others in your trust are using so that co-ordinated surveys can be carried out in each department or practice. If they are, ensure that your own results can be differentiated if you want to use the results for your own development, and do not just present those of your team or service as a whole.

Evaluation of consent issues to look at how you deal with, or pass on, information to others

Patients should feel free to decline investigations, treatment, preventative measures, etc. without feeling that this will prejudice the quality of the care they receive in future. Consent is only meaningful if someone understands the explanation and implications of participating. For instance, you should explain why you are carrying out a survey and whether participating in it could lead to them being asked to co-operate with more in-depth work at a later time.

The right to grant or withhold consent presupposes the person's mental capacity or ability to do so. There is an association between someone's competency or capacity to be well informed and the extent of their previous education. You should be aware of this and act accordingly by recognising the inability of some individuals to provide informed consent when they have educational, social, language and cultural reasons that limit their understanding of complex issues.

You might establish the extent to which patients whose consent you have obtained felt that you had informed them of the various options. You might ask relevant patients for feedback using a semi-structured interview schedule that you and an independent colleague have previously agreed. Ten such patients should give you a fair idea. You might examine the probity issues of consent in any research you are involved with, or when financial or commercial pressures exist.

Providing evidence of your competence and performance

You must be able to demonstrate how you meet standards expected of you as a practising midwife with a record of your performance in your personal professional or revalidation portfolio if you want to retain a licence to practise. Although the final requirements for revalidation are not yet known, you should continue to gather evidence of your performance around key areas – for example those expected for doctors[84] which are all relevant to midwives.

1 Good clinical care relates to providing clinical care, supporting self care, keeping records (including writing reports and keeping colleagues informed), access and availability, patient safety, treatment in emergencies and providing effective treatments based on the best available evidence.
2 Maintaining good clinical practice includes keeping up to date, maintaining and improving your performance.
3 Relationships with patients emphasises the good midwife–patient partnership: providing patients with information about your services, maintaining trust and good communication, respecting patients' privacy and right to confidentiality, obtaining consent, avoiding discrimination and prejudice, relating well to patients and being open and honest if things go wrong.
4 Working with colleagues describes your work within teams, protecting patients from harm, respecting colleagues, arranging cover, referring patients and delegation.
5 Teaching and training, appraising and assessing relates to teaching or training colleagues or students; appraising or assessing peers, employees or students.
6 Probity is about being honest and trustworthy and acting with integrity – e.g. in writing reports, financial and commercial dealings, conducting research in an ethical manner, being open about conflicts of interest and supplying references.
7 Health can include how you overcome or minimise health problems in yourself, or help with or address health problems in other midwives.

Essentially competence is being able to perform the tasks and roles required of a midwife in your post to the expected standard.[85] Competencies can be described as a combination of knowledge, skills and attitudes – relevant to how you do your job. You may have a competency-based job description which defines those competencies central to your effective performance at work in that role. In a wider sense, 'competence' to carry out an entire role consists of having all the individual competences required, plus the ability to use judgement at a higher level (for example by knowing when to use which competence and when it is clinically right to depart from a standard clinical approach).

There is an important difference between knowing what to do (competence) and actually doing it (performance). A **competent** midwife knows how to administer drugs safely, but might sometimes fail to do so; a midwife who **performs** adequately always works in a safe way. Revalidation is relevant to patient safety as it tests performance as well as competence.

The steps of the evidence cycle for demonstrating your standards of practice or competence and any necessary improvements are shown in Figure 7. This learning cycle can be applied to all components of your job. Although the five steps are shown in sequence here you would expect to move backwards and forwards from step to step, because of new information, a change in circumstances or a modification of your earlier ideas. New information might accrue when research is published which affects your clinical behaviour or standards; or a critical incident or patient complaint might occur which causes you and others to think anew about your standards or the way that services are delivered. The arrows in Figure 7 show that you might re-set your target or aspirations for good practice having undertaken exercises to identify what you need to learn or determine what, or if, there are gaps in service delivery.

We suggest that you demonstrate your competence in focused areas of your day-to-day work by completing several cycles of evidence drawn from a variety of clinical or other areas each year.

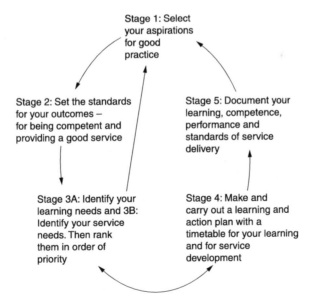

Figure 7:   Steps of the evidence cycle.

As you start to collate information about this five stage cycle, discuss any problems about the standards of care or services you are looking at, with colleagues, experts in this area, clinical tutors, etc. You should develop a wide range and depth of evidence so that you can show that you are competent in your day-to-day general work as well as for any special areas of expertise or diverse settings.

You should be able to demonstrate that you can maintain a satisfactory standard of clinical care most of the time in your everyday work. Some of the time you will be brilliant, of course! Celebrate those moments. On other occasions, you or others will be critical of your performance and feel that you could have done much better. Reflect on those episodes to learn from them.

Step 1 Select your aspirations for good practice

By adopting or adapting descriptions of what an 'excellent' midwife should be aiming for, you are defining the standards of practice for which all midwives should be aiming. Your definition of excellence might be about being 'consistently good'.

This consistency is a critical factor in considering competence and performance too. The documents that you collect in your evidence cycles must reflect consistency over time and in different circumstances, for example with various types of patients or your practice at different times of day. This will show that you have not only performed well on one occasion or for one type of baseline assessment, but also sustained your performance over time and under different conditions.

Step 2 Set the standards of your outcomes – for being competent and providing a good service

Outcomes might include:

- the way that you apply your learning
- a skill you have learnt or refined
- a protocol you have developed and/or applied
- a strategy that is implemented
- meeting of recommended standards.

The level at which you should be performing at work depends on your particular field of expertise. Community midwives are good at seeing the wider picture, whilst hospital midwives might be expert in a narrower specialism, so that the level of competence expected for a clinical area will vary depending on the midwife's role and responsibilities. You would not, for example, expect midwives based mainly in the labour suite to be competent at completing a full obstetric and social history (although some may be) as you would a midwife working primarily in the community. You would expect both to recognise the limits of their competence and to refer to a colleague with more expertise when appropriate.

You could incorporate those components specified by universities for their postgraduate awards into your standards or outcomes. The national Masters Framework consists of eight components that shape the individual postgraduate award programme outcomes and the learning outcomes of individual modules for the postgraduate awards. You could document your professional development to date in a form that can be readily 'Accredited for Prior Experiential Learning' (APEL) by universities (contact your local universities if you want more information about this process). You might then be given credits for learning against an intended postgraduate award. It would save you from duplicating work as well as speeding your progress through the award.

If you have information or data about your practice showing that it was sub-standard or that you were not competent, you might want to exclude that from your portfolio. However, it is better to include everything of relevance, then go on to demonstrate how you addressed the gaps in your performance and made sustained improvements.

Remember to protect the confidentiality of patients and colleagues when you collect data.

Step 3 Identify your learning and service needs and rank them in order of priority

The type and depth of documentation you need to gather will cover:

- the context in which you work
- your knowledge and skills in relation to any particular role or responsibility of your current post.

You may decide to use a few selected methods to identify your learning and service development needs. For this type of combined assessment, you might use a variety of tools such as:

- a self-assessment using a rating scale to assess your skills and attitudes, or peer review
- a SWOT (strengths, weaknesses, opportunities and threats) analysis
- patient feedback or patient satisfaction surveys

- significant event audit, constructive feedback with peer observation, multi-source (360°) feedback
- identifying team difficulties to recognise where a lack of competence, accessibility or use of resources has affected the process or outcome for a patient
- challenges during teaching and training to justify why you do what you do
- looking at how you deal with issues of consent for examination, investigation or treatment and if patients' autonomy and right to decline is respected
- audit of protocols and guidelines, checking how well procedures are followed; reviews of how resources, access and availability were managed
- case review of patient records.

Your learning needs should take into account your aspirations for the future too – personal or career development for you, or improvements in the way you deliver patient care.

Group and summarise your learning and service development needs from the exercises you have carried out. Grade them according to the priority you set. You may put one at a higher priority because it fits in with service development needs established in the strategic and operational plans of your trust, primary care organisation or practice, or vice versa. If you have identified a service development need by several different methods of assessment or with several different patient groups or clinical conditions, then it will have a higher priority than something only identified once.

Look back at your aspirations and standards set out in Steps 1 and 2. Match your learning or service development needs with one or more of these standards, or others that you have set yourself.

Step 4 Make and carry out a learning and action plan with a timetable for your personal and service development

In the unlikely event that you have not identified any learning needs for yourself or the service as a whole, you could tidy up the presentation of your evidence for inclusion in your portfolio as at the end of Step 5. However, it would be preferable to undertake more learning and service need assessments over a wider range of your work or anticipated future roles.

Think about whether:

- you have defined your learning objectives sufficiently – what you need to learn to be able to attain the standards and outcomes you have described in Step 2

- you can justify spending time and effort on the topics you prioritised in Step 3. Is the topic important enough to your work, the NHS as a whole or patient safety? Does the clinical or non-clinical event occur sufficiently often to warrant time and effort spent?
- the time and resources for learning about that topic or making the associated improvements to service delivery are available. Check that you are not trying to do too much too quickly, or you will become discouraged
- learning about that topic will make a difference to the care you or others can provide for patients
- one particular topic fits in with other areas you have identified as needing to learn more about
- you have achieved a good balance across your areas of work or between your personal aspirations and the basic requirements of the service.

Decide on what method(s) of learning is most appropriate for your task or role or the standards you are expecting to attain or sustain.

Describe how you will carry out your learning tasks and what you will do by a specified time. Note down how you will apply your learning and how and when it will be evaluated. Build in some milestones so that you do not suddenly get to the end of 12 months and discover that you have only done half of your plan.

Your action plan should also include your role or responsibilities in remedying any gaps in service delivery that you identified in Step 3.

Step 5 Document your learning, competence, performance and standards of service delivery

You might choose to document that you have attained your defined outcomes by repeating the learning and service needs assessments that you started with. You could record your increased confidence and competence in dealing with situations that you previously avoided or performed inadequately, your increased range of knowledge and skills, or improvements to patient care.

Why not aim for four or five cycles of evidence per year, linked to key areas in your specialty from different domains?

Example cycles of evidence of your competence and performance

Evidence cycle 1: preserving confidentiality

Focus on confidentiality; teaching and training.

Case study 1

It is the first time you have had student nurses placed with you and you want to ensure that they are aware of the professional guidelines on confidentiality and teach them about the importance of making sure that young people understand the code of confidentiality whilst they are on their placement with you.

Step 1 Set your aspirations for good practice. The excellent midwife:

- maintains the confidentiality of patient specific information
- ensures that patients are aware of when they are receiving care from students and are not put at risk.

Step 2 Set the standards for your outcomes:

- all members of the team including you, new members of staff and students are familiar with guidelines for confidentiality in relation to patients receiving healthcare.

Step 3A Identify your learning needs:

- assess your knowledge about the limits of confidentiality, e.g. for providing care to under-16 year olds
- ask a colleague who has teaching experience how you could best approach an in-house training session on maintaining confidentiality for teenagers of different ages that will convey the most important messages and lead to changes where necessary.

Step 3B Identify your service needs:

- compare the protocol for confidentiality with guidelines in the *Confidentiality and Young People* toolkit[86]
- review the intended induction programme for new members of staff, including administrative staff and students on placement to assess the extent to which knowledge of confidentiality features and is addressed.

Step 4 Make and carry out a learning and action plan:

- talk to practice educators about how to undertake learning needs assessments of others from different disciplines with different levels of responsibilities in respect of confidentiality
- prepare for and run an interactive teaching session on confidentiality for patients of all age groups with special focus on teenagers. You might invite the whole team, including students, community midwives, family planning or school nurses, etc. You could use the *Confidentiality and Young People*

toolkit for promoting discussion with the team at the session. You use a quiz before and after the session to evaluate the effectiveness of the session.

Step 5 Document your learning, competence, performance and standards of service delivery:

- include the results from the quiz completed by those attending teaching session before and after training about confidentiality
- keep an incident record kept by the team of any reported or perceived breaches of confidentiality by any one working in, or associated with, the practice
- record the existence of personal learning plans based on learning needs assessments for new staff by end of their induction period
- include in your records the revised protocol in line with the *Confidentiality and Young People* toolkit.

Case study 1 continued

Other staff colleagues join your teaching session with the students using the video from the *Confidentiality and Young People* toolkit. All get full marks in the quiz after watching the video.

Evidence cycle 2: learning from complaints

Focus on complaints; working with colleagues.

Case study 2 Complaints management

The clinic where you work has received a patient complaint about lack of privacy for patients when attending for antenatal care. This has prompted you all as a team to review the way that your complaints system functions.

Step 1 Set your aspirations for good practice. The excellent midwife:

- is not afraid of complaints, recognising that they can have positive outcomes of improving future ways of working
- apologises appropriately when things go wrong, and has an adequate complaints procedure in place.

Step 2 Set the standards or your outcomes:

- have effective processes for preventing the need for, and managing, complaints from patients.

Step 3A Identify your learning needs:

- examine as a significant event one or more complaints, e.g. where patients have not been made aware of the complaints process
- compare the actual care of a patient against an acceptable standard of care for a range of clinical conditions as part of an ongoing review for a clinical area that has been the subject of a complaint (e.g. privacy given to patients as in the case study). You could use peer review by asking respected colleagues or compare yourselves against a published standard such as a guideline by a responsible body of professional opinion.

Step 3B Identify your service needs:

- audit patient complaints in the preceding 12 months: the number, the outcomes and how the complaint system is advertised, etc.
- audit the extent to which midwives are following agreed protocols. This shows how well being proactive about prevents or minimises the likelihood of the source of the complaint recurring
- audit vulnerable areas. Look back at the analysis of complaints to identify useful areas for focusing learning, e.g. a review of the method of informing patients of the results of their blood test results.

Step 4 Make and carry out a learning and action plan:

- ask your trust to look at the complaints system and feed back how it can be improved (if at all)
- arrange a tutorial with midwifery colleagues and managers to discuss preventing and managing complaints
- undertake reflection of critical incidents including how to share the information with the team and respond as a team.

Step 5 Document your learning, competence, performance and standards of service delivery:

- collect evidence of clinical competence for all staff to guard against a complaint
- keep a copy of the protocol of the patient complaint process against which consecutive complaints can be audited in another 12 months' time
- document guidance about physical examinations including that the reason for any examination should be communicated clearly, that a chaperone should be offered for any internal or breast examination, and the comfort and privacy of the patient should always be paramount to avoid potential complaints
- ensure that a file containing practice protocols is available for easy reference (e.g. on the desktop of the computer).

Case study 2 continued

You are invited by your trust to take part in advising other departments about the handling of complaints because they were impressed by the way your complaint system was applied when you discussed this in a staff meeting.

Evidence cycle 3: good preventive care

Focus on clinical care; smoking cessation.

Case study 3

Miss Flower has just had her first baby. At five pounds the baby was small for a full-term baby. Miss Flower is a smoker and she tells you that apart from the midwife mentioning that she should stop smoking when she first booked in for her pregnancy, no one else has ever advised her to stop smoking in the past when she has come for contraceptive or other healthcare.

Step 1 Set your aspirations for good practice. The excellent midwife has:

- a structured approach for undertaking preventive care
- all pregnant women who smoke are offered advice about the risks of smoking and the benefits of quitting and further support and help.

Step 2 Set the standards for your outcomes:

- every patient attending for antenatal in first trimester is asked if they smoke and has their smoking history recorded.

Step 3A Identify your learning needs:

- self-assess your knowledge of magnitude and nature of health risks associated with pregnant women who are smokers.

Step 3B Identify your service needs:

- carry out a patient survey: ask 10 consecutive patients who smoke (who are in the last trimester of pregnancy) if they have received advice about smoking within the last two years, and if so, how appropriate the advice was perceived to be, when it had been given and by whom
- audit the smoking status of patients attending antenatal care in the last trimester for: existence of record of smoking status, extent of advice and support or help offered; carry out second audit focusing on changes in smoking behaviour at the postnatal appointment

- carry out a significant event audit of cases of babies born to mothers who smoke who have health problems that might be associated with mother's smoking status, e.g. low birth weight.

Step 4 Make and carry out a learning and action plan:

- read up about risks of smoking and provision of best practice in motivating people to stop smoking
- talk to smokers at an informal group, e.g. in the waiting room during an antenatal clinic, and actively listen to their feedback about improving services and the quality and extent of the advice they have received about stopping smoking
- audiotape (with the patient's informed consent) a consultation (or two) where you give advice to a patient who is a smoker, offer them further help and try to motivate them to stop. Ask a health promotion expert to comment on your approach and give targeted feedback to you about your knowledge, skills and attitudes.

Step 5 Document your learning, competence, performance and standards of service delivery:

- keep the surveys of smokers – two separate cohorts of patients at different time periods before and after putting your learning and action plan into practice, or one cohort of the same patients surveyed twice over time
- keep a copy of the practice protocol relating to smoking cessation
- carry out a re-audit of the recording in antenatal patients' notes of smoking status, extent of advice and support or help offered, and the change of smoking behaviour at follow-up.

Case study 3 continued

Miss Flower's baby thrives as she makes up her mind not to inflict passive smoking on her baby or her partner at home. She quits after only using nicotine replacement therapy for a month and had not resumed smoking 12 months later.

Evidence cycle 4: management responsibilities

Focus on management; committee work.

Case study 4

As a midwifery team leader, you are required to attend the monthly directorate meeting both as a member of the directorate and to report on developments and needs in your specialised area.

Step 1 The excellent midwife:

- attends as many meetings each year as possible
- is aware of current issues facing the trust/directorate/practice
- is aware of overall organisational strategy
- ensures that they chair meetings effectively, the committee has the correct structure, and meetings are convenient.

Step 2 Set standards for your outcomes:

- attend essential committee meetings regularly
- send apologies if you cannot attend
- read the minutes of the previous meeting checking for errors and that tasks that were designated to you have been completed
- prepare regular reports on your particular areas of interest or responsibility and circulate papers in good time for the meeting
- review attendance if chairing committee; ensure that the meeting does not usually over-run.

Step 3A Identify your learning needs:

- read trust and DH policy documents so as to be well briefed; identify gaps in knowledge
- develop options for solutions at the same time as presenting any problems.

Step 3B Identify your service needs:

- determine if sufficient time to prepare for and attend the meeting
- get feedback from colleagues as to how well you presented your case
- if you chaired the meeting, get feedback on how effectively this was done.

Step 4 Make and carry out a learning and action plan:

- observe how others chair meetings, prepare reports, present information, effect agreement among colleagues and achieve required outcomes
- attend a course on time-management
- attend a course on effecting change in an organisation
- attend a course or read up on chairing meetings and group interactions.

Step 5 Document your learning, competence, performance and standards of service delivery:

- keep records of your attendance
- write a summary of the meetings and reflect on your performance
- keep a record of your achievements
- keep a record of strategy documents and project progress.

Case study 4 continued

Having addressed the above issues, you find that you are far more effective in the meeting and can develop service aspirations more readily.

Evidence cycle 5: minimising risks to maternity patients

Focus on staff management; service development.

Case study 5

As a midwifery team leader you welcome two novice midwives who have commenced their first placements on the labour ward suite and need to gain and maintain their skills to manage a range of obstetric emergencies; these include shoulder dystocia, vaginal breech birth, postpartum haemorrhage, cord prolapse, maternal and neonatal resuscitation. You are aware that the hospital trust has not replaced midwifery staff as they leave their jobs, to make savings for the hospital budget. Your midwifery colleagues are finding it increasingly difficult to provide effective care to individual women and babies because of their heavy caseloads. You believe that staff shortages mean increased risks to patient safety. You are worried about whether there will always be a senior midwife available to supervise your new starters, whilst they gain experience and expertise in basic and complex cases.

Step 1 The excellent midwife:

- has the knowledge and skills to manage an obstetric emergency to be able to provide safe and effective care
- provides clinical supervision for junior midwifery staff as appropriate to their knowledge and skills; and the complexity of the case
- identifies risks to patient care arising from the work environment and reports those outside their control to senior management for their action.

Step 2 Set standards for your outcomes:

- experienced midwives provide effective clinical supervision for inexperienced midwives so that risks to patient safety are minimised; and there is an experienced midwife involved in every maternity patient's care at all times
- review of the outcome of each obstetric emergency demonstrates that the midwives providing care had sufficient knowledge and skills, and that junior staff were supervised by experienced midwives

- risk factors and gaps in care are identified by routine review of each obstetric emergency; these are reported to senior management who take appropriate action to minimise the chance of recurrence.

Step 3A Identify your learning needs:

- reflect on your knowledge and skills in managing obstetric emergencies; draw upon any departmental reviews of recent emergencies where you played a role
- undertake a significant event audit of an obstetric emergency which had one or more negative outcomes, where you were supervising the junior midwife with a substantial caring role in that case; you lead the team meeting, discussing and reviewing the case. Divide the learning points between those concerning professional development, extent and nature of clinical supervision, and service issues such as inadequate resources.

Step 3B Identify your service needs:

- undertake a team activity to review staffing levels (including capacity for clinical supervision of inexperienced staff; experts on call for neonatal emergencies) over previous four weeks as well as relevant to any obstetric emergency cases, location and availability of emergency drugs and equipment. Include personal accounts from team members as well as hospital staffing records
- undertake SWOT analysis as a team to review capability and capacity for coping with obstetric emergencies throughout 24-hour periods
- look at the hospital's risk assurance framework for the previous year; note what entries have been made in relation to capacity and capability in responding to obstetric emergencies; find out what actions have been taken and if intended improvements have been evaluated
- consider the clinical supervision policy; run an audit to check how the policy is working in practice.

Step 4 Make and carry out a learning and action plan:

- participating in the discussion of the significant event audit and drawing up an action plan after the SWOT analysis will generate informal learning
- arrange a tutorial with the hospital's risk manager to better understand the risk assurance framework and how to complete it so that the senior managers note and address concerns about potential risks associated with low staffing levels and threats to patient safety
- visit one or more hospitals to see how their clinical supervision arrangements work out in practice; discuss and agree revisions to your policy
- visit one or more obstetric units in other hospitals to see how they handle emergencies, their staffing levels, their equipment, etc.

Step 5 Document your learning, competence, performance and standards of service delivery:

- keep records of the reviews, audit, significant event audit, SWOT analysis and actions agreed and completed
- include revised clinical supervision policy
- document the continuing discussions with senior management about review of staffing levels, actions addressing identified risks to patient safety from your reviews and benchmarking against other hospital units.

Case study 5 continued

Senior management realised that midwifery staffing levels were critically low, generating unacceptable risks to patient safety and rendering the revised clinical supervision policy untenable. The hospital focused on embedding more quality indicators in their productivity calculations in relation to the obstetric services they provided; and as a result recruited additional midwifery staff. This in turn provided more experienced midwives to supervise and support midwives starting out in their careers.

EVALUATE YOUR NEWLY GAINED KNOWLEDGE AND SKILLS IN CLINICAL EFFECTIVENESS AND CLINICAL GOVERNANCE

Evaluate how much you have learned by doing this programme and compare your answers to questions 1 and 2 below with the equivalent questions in your initial self-assessment of your knowledge and skills about the topic at the beginning of this book.

Please circle as many answers as apply or fill in the information requested.

1 How confident do you feel *now* that you know enough about clinical effectiveness to be able to:

Ask a relevant question?	*Very*	*Somewhat*	*Not at all*
Undertake a search of the literature?	*Very*	*Somewhat*	*Not at all*
Find readily available evidence?	*Very*	*Somewhat*	*Not at all*
Weigh up available evidence?	*Very*	*Somewhat*	*Not at all*
Decide if changes in practice are warranted?	*Very*	*Somewhat*	*Not at all*
Make changes in practice as appropriate?	*Very*	*Somewhat*	*Not at all*

2 Which database(s) have you used in this programme?

Medline   Cochrane   OMNI   Other (what?)

3 What level of evidence did you find in answer to your question (or main question if you posed more than one question)?

Strong evidence from at least one systematic review of multiple, well-designed randomised controlled trials (RCTs).

Strong evidence from at least one properly designed RCT of appropriate size.

Evidence from well-designed trials without randomisation.

Evidence from well-designed non-experimental studies from more than one centre or research group.

Opinions of well-respected authorities, based on clinical evidence, descriptive studies or reports of expert committees.

No evidence at all.

4 To whom have you given a report about the evidence you found?
   Colleagues at work   Friends/family   Bosses (managers) at work
   Other (who?)

5 What is/are the outcome(s) of you asking your main question and finding
   the evidence?

   Made change(s) to an aspect of work – if so, please describe what change(s) you
   have made or plan to make, who was involved in deciding to make the
   change(s), who is involved in the new change(s), whether you need any
   more resources or training and how you will review the change(s):

   Decided against making any change(s) to any aspect of work – if so, why did you
   decide not to make any change(s) and who was involved in that decision?

   Other outcome – what?

6 How will you use your new-found knowledge about clinical effectiveness in
   the future?

(Hopefully, your own response will reflect the position that everyone working in the NHS is responsible for the quality of care their team provides.)

7 You have just been appointed as the clinical governance lead in your workplace. What are your roles and responsibilities likely to be and how will you go about promoting a positive culture of clinical governance among your team members?

Write down your answers – you can glean the information you need from Stage 6, which is the chapter on applying clinical governance in practice.

USEFUL PUBLICATIONS OF EVIDENCE ALREADY AVAILABLE

Some evidence is already available, so it is not necessary to appraise all the evidence yourself. The following resources will be useful.

Bandolier provides key evidence about the effectiveness of healthcare, reviewing national and international evidence. It is available by personal subscription. It is available in full text on the Internet at www.ebandolier.com

Clinical Evidence is a compendium of evidence on the effects of common clinical interventions, published by the BMJ Publishing Group. It is updated and expanded every six months and summarises the best available evidence about the prevention and treatment of a wide range of clinical conditions such as nausea and vomiting in pregnancy, pre-eclampsia and postnatal depression. A plus point is that its contents are driven by questions rather than by the availability of research evidence and so it identifies gaps in the evidence, leaving you to make your own decisions. *Clinical Evidence* is freely available to all, www.clinicalevidence.com/ceweb/conditions/index.jsp

Clinical Governance Bulletin is a bimonthly publication from the Royal Society of Medicine Press to which institutions and individuals can subscribe. The contents report and review quality aspects of local initiatives in primary and secondary healthcare. The Bulletin has an emphasis on practical 'how we did it' material. It is distributed free to some NHS professionals with financial support from The Health Foundation. Full text is online at www.rsmpress. co.uk/cgb.htm

Drug & Therapeutics Bulletin (DTB) is published monthly and provides independent evaluations of drugs and other medical treatments and management issues. See www.dtb.org.uk/

In May 2006, the Department of Health withdrew the funding for free provision of DTB for the NHS. You may still have access via an Athens password: check with your healthcare library.

Evidence-Based Medicine provides critical appraisals of systematic reviews and primary research, with a commentary from a clinical expert. Much of the journal content is available as part of the Evidence Based Medicine Reviews (EBMR) database by subscription from OVID at www.ovid.com/site/catalog/

Database/904.jsp?top=2&mid=3&bottom=7&subsection=10 Print subscriptions are available from the BMJ Publishing Group, BMA House, Tavistock Square, London WC1H 9JR. See www.ebm.bmj.com

HSTAT (Health Services/Technology Assessment Text) Free full text guidelines and summaries of the systematic reviews on which they are based. See www.ncbi.nlm.nih.gov/books/bv.fcgi?rid=hstat

MeReC Publications produces several publications – *MeReC Bulletin, MeReC Extra, MeReC Briefing* and *MeReC Rapid Review. MeReC Bulletin* focuses on clinical and therapeutic topics. *MeReC Extra* provides brief updates and overviews on recent key issues, questions and controversies. *MeReC Briefing* provided an in-depth overview of some of the major issues, trials and clinical papers. It was discontinued in 2006, but back copies are still available. *MeReC Rapid Review* provides a quick appraisal of the evidence, in the context of the current evidence base. This portfolio of publications provides concise, evidence-based information about medicines and prescribing-related issues. They are freely available at: www.npc.co.uk/merec.htm

Netting the Evidence provides an evidence-based virtual library and is the closest thing on the Web to a 'one-stop shop' for evidence-based healthcare. See www.shef.ac.uk/scharr/ir/netting

Organisations

Aggressive Research Intelligence Facility (ARIF)
ARIF is a specialist unit that aims to improve the incorporation of research findings into population-level healthcare decisions in the NHS by helping healthcare workers access and interpret research evidence, particularly systematic reviews of research. The website provides summaries of the research information ARIF has uncovered in response to requests received. You can submit your own questions. The website is at: www.arif.bham.ac.uk

Centre for Reviews and Dissemination (CRD)
CRD is a sibling organisation of the UK Cochrane Centre, funded by the Department of Health to provide information on the effectiveness and cost-effectiveness of treatments and the delivery and organisation of healthcare. CRD carries out systematic reviews, provides a database of good quality reviews, offers a dissemination and information service and helps to promote research-based practice in the NHS. CRD plays an important role in disseminating the contents of Cochrane reviews to NHS decision makers. It provides an information and enquiry service on reviews and economic evaluations for

healthcare professionals, purchasers and providers, NHS managers, information providers, health service researchers and consumer organisations. Its main outputs are: Database of Abstracts of Reviews of Effects (DARE); NHS Economic Evaluation Database (NHSEED); and the Health Technology Assessment (HTA) Database. Centre for Reviews and Dissemination, University of York, York Y10 5DD. Tel: 01904 321040. Email: crd@york.ac.uk The website is at: www.york.ac.uk/inst/crd/

National Institute for Health and Clinical Excellence (NICE) is an independent organisation that provides national guidance on promoting good health and preventing and treating ill health. They have published clinical guidelines on gynaecology, pregnancy and birth including:

- caesarean section
- induction of labour
- antenatal and postnatal mental health
- antenatal care
- postnatal care
- fertility
- heavy menstrual bleeding
- long-acting reversible contraception.

In addition to guidelines for health professionals, NICE also produce guidelines for patients, carers and the public. NICE also provides tools to help health professionals implement NICE guidelines. For more details see: www.nice.org.uk/

The NHS Clinical Governance Support Team (CGST) is a learning organisation that aims to support clinical and non-clinical healthcare workers to keep their 'eyes on the prize' by providing high-quality, safe, patient-centred healthcare that is accountable, systematic and sustainable. See www.cgsupport.nhs.uk/

NHS Quality Improvement Clinical Effectiveness Co-ordination Unit. NHS Quality Improvement Scotland (NHS QIS) is made up of a number of specialist units that work together to improve the quality of healthcare delivered by NHS Scotland. The Clinical Effectiveness Co-ordination Unit commissions clinical guidelines from SIGN and other bodies to develop a strategy for clinical effectiveness/audit and commission programmes and projects to put it into effect, and liaises with NICE to secure appropriate Scottish input to its work and dissemination of its output to NHS Scotland. For more information see: www.nhshealthquality.org/nhsqis/2038.html#1

The Royal College of Obstetricians and Gynaecologists (RCOG) has developed the following documents to assist Fellows and Members in discharging their clinical responsibilities: audit, improving patient safety, risk management for maternity and gynaecology, obtaining valid consent, producing a clinical practice guideline, patient involvement in enhancing service provision, and searching for evidence. For more details see: www.rcog.org.uk/index.asp?PageID=2

Useful websites

British Medical Association (BMA) library specialises in clinical medicine, medical ethics, clinical governance and social and political issues. The Royal College of Midwives (RCM) library is an institutional member and can obtain material from the BMA library for members. The library runs training courses for health professionals in literature searching and critical appraisal. www.bma.org.uk/ap.nsf/Content/HubTLlibraryandmedline

Centre for Evidence-Based Medicine (CEBM) promotes evidence-based healthcare via workshops, resources, research tools and educational materials for health professionals. www.cebm.net/

Contact, Help, Advice and Information Networks (CHAIN) are online networks for people working in health and social care that provide informal, multiprofessional and cross organisational ways of contacting people to exchange ideas and share knowledge on particular areas of interest. http://chain.ulcc.ac.uk/chain/index.html

Department of Health (DH) publications: many DH documents are downloadable. www.dh.gov.uk/en/Publicationsandstatistics/index.htm

Geneva Foundation for Medical Research gives a comprehensive and useful list of links to guidelines, reviews, position statements, recommendations, and standards in obstetrics, gynaecology and reproductive medicine. www.gfmer.ch/Guidelines/Obstetrics_gynecology_guidelines.php

Internet for Nursing, Midwifery and Health Visiting: a virtual training suite series of internet tutorials. www.vts.intute.ac.uk/he/tutorial/nurse

Intute: Health and Life Sciences: a free online service providing access to web resources for education and research. www.intute.ac.uk/healthandlifesciences/

MIDIRS: a bibliographic database that includes leaflets, events, news, online bookshop and comprehensive list of links. www.midirs.org

Midwives Online: a commercial site for midwives and for expectant and new parents. www.midwivesonline.com/

Nursing and Midwifery Council (NMC): the regulatory body for the nursing professions within the UK. Provides an advice sheet on clinical governance and many of its publications are downloadable free of charge. www.nmc-uk.org

National Library for Health (NLH): a single search facility that allows simultaneous searching across multiple resources. The RCM is collaborating on the development of a 'specialist library' for women's health. www.library. nhs.uk

Netting the Evidence facilitates evidence-based healthcare by providing support and access to organisations and learning resources such as software, journals and an evidence-based virtual library. www.shef.ac.uk/scharr/ir/ netting

Primary Care Electronic Library (PCEL) has indexed and classified over 1000 internet sites relevant to primary care. www.pcel.info/index.php

Social Care Institute for Excellence (SCIE) has a role to develop and promote knowledge about good practice in social care. It has a bibliographic database, Social Care Online (formerly CareData), a directory of research in social care and a wide range of freely-downloadable reports and other documents. www.scie.org.uk

Trawling the Net signposts free internet databases that might be of interest to NHS staff. www.shef.ac.uk/scharr/ir/trawling.html

TRIP Database allows health professionals access to evidence. www. tripdatabase.com/index.html

WeBNF: a searchable, electronic, full-text version of the British National Formulary which provides clear, concise and understandable information on the selection and use of medicines available in the UK. http://bnf.org/

Virginia Henderson International Nursing Library: provides access to research and conference abstracts. Researchers can also submit up-to-date research findings. www.nursinglibrary.org

Further reading

- Baker M, Maskrey N, Kirk S. *Clinical Effectiveness and Primary Care*. Oxford: Radcliffe Medical Press; 1997 (out of print).
- Campbell P, Longbottom A, Pooler A. *Nursing in General Practice: the toolkit for nurses and health care assistants*. Oxford: Radcliffe Publishing; 2007.
- Chambers R, Boath E, Rogers D. *Clinical Effectiveness and Clinical Governance Made Easy*. 4th ed. Oxford: Radcliffe Publishing; 2007.
- Chambers R, Wakley G. *Making Clinical Governance Work for You*. Oxford: Radcliffe Medical Press; 2000.
- Craig JV, Smyth RL. *The Evidence-based Practice Manual for Nurses*. 2nd ed. Edinburgh: Churchill Livingstone; 2007.
- Crombie IK. *The Pocket Guide to Critical Appraisal*. London: BMJ Publishing Group; 1996.
- Department of Health. *Achieving Effective Practice: a clinical effectiveness and research information pack for nurses, midwives and health visitors*. London: DH; 2007. www.dh.gov.uk/assetRoot/04/04/24/62/04042462.pdf or www.intute.ac.uk/healthandlifesciences/cgi-bin/fullrecord.pl?handle=20261833
- Dunning M *et al*. *Turning Evidence into Everyday Practice*. London: The King's Fund; 1998.
- Greenhalgh T. *How to Read a Paper: the basics of evidence-based medicine*. 3rd ed. Oxford: Blackwell; 2006.
- The Information Centre: Information Catalogue www.ic.nhs.uk/
- Jones R, Kinmonth AL (eds). *Critical Reading for Primary Care*. Oxford: Oxford University Press; 1995.
- Kobelt G. *Health Economics: an introduction to economic evaluation*. 2nd ed. London: Office of Health Economics; 2002.
- Lennox A, Bonser W, Robinson D, Muneer M. *A Practical Guide for Involving the Public in Health and Social Care Services*. Leicester: Leicester Promotions; 2004.
- McSherry R, Pearce P. *Clinical Governance: a guide to implementation for healthcare professionals*. 2nd ed. Oxford: Blackwell Publishing; 2007.
- Muir Gray JA. *Evidence-Based Healthcare*. 2nd ed. Edinburgh: Churchill Livingstone; 2001.
- Ridsdale L. *Evidence-Based General Practice: a critical reader*. London: Saunders; 1995.
- Sackett D, Strauss S, Richardson S *et al*. *Evidence-Based Medicine: how to practice and teach EBM*. 2nd ed. Edinburgh: Churchill Livingstone; 2000.
- Sale DNT. *Understanding Clinical Governance and Quality Assurance: making it happen*. Basingstoke: Palgrave Macmillan; 2005.
- Scottish Executive. *Making Choices, Facing Challenges: developing your research career in nursing, midwifery and the allied health professions*. NHS

Education for Scotland; 2005. www.scotland.gov.uk/Publications/2005/02/20730/53067
- Swage T. *Clinical Governance in Healthcare Practice*. 2nd ed. Oxford: Butterworth-Heinemann; 2003.
- van Zwanenberg T, Harrison J (eds). *Clinical Governance in Primary Care*. 2nd ed. Oxford: Radcliffe Medical Press; 2004.

REFERENCES

1 NHS Executive. *Promoting Clinical Effectiveness*. London: NHS Executive; 1996.

2 Hicks N. Evidence-based health care. *Bandolier* 1997; **4(5)**: 8.

3 Sackett DL, Rosenberg WM, Muir Gray JA *et al*. Evidence based medicine: what it is and what it isn't. *BMJ* 1996; **312**: 71–2.

4 Haynes RB, Sackett DL, Muir Gray JA *et al*. Transferring evidence from research into practice: 1. The role of clinical care research evidence in clinical decisions. *Evid Based Med* 1996; **1(7)**: 196–7.

5 Haynes RB, Sackett DL, Cook DJ *et al*. Transferring evidence from research into practice: 4. Overcoming barriers to application. *Evid Based Med* 1997; **2(3)**: 68–9.

6 Dunning M, Abi-Aad G, Gilbert D *et al*. *Turning Evidence into Everyday Practice*. London: King's Fund; 1997.

7 Andrews S. A framework for evaluation of scientific research papers. *Midwives* 2007; **9(8)**: 306–9.

8 Lyndon-Rochelle M, Hodnett E, Renfrew M *et al*. A systematic approach for midwifery students. *MIDIRS Midwifery Digest* 2003; **13(4)**: 454–5.

9 Hancock H. Evidence based midwifery practice in Australian rural and remote settings: an unknown entity. *Evidence Based Midwifery* 2006; **4**: 131–4.

10 Paterson C. Problem setting and problem solving: the role of evidence-based medicine. *J Roy Soc Med* 1997; **90**: 304–6.

11 Hughes J, Humphrey C, Rogers S *et al*. *Evidence into Action: changing practice in primary care*. Occasional Paper 84. London: Royal College of General Practitioners; 2002.

12 Department of Health. *Coronary Heart Disease. National Service Frameworks*. London: Department of Health; 2000.

13 National Institute for Clinical Excellence. *Compilation. Summary of Guidance issued to the NHS in England and Wales*. Issue 10. London: National Institute for Clinical Excellence; 2005. www.nice.org.uk

14 Black N. Evidence based policy: proceed with care. *BMJ* 2001; **323**: 275–9.

15 Royal College of General Practitioners. *Portfolio-based Learning in General Practice: a report of a working group on higher professional education*. Occasional Paper 63. London: RCGP; 1993.

16 Treasure W. Portfolio-based learning pilot scheme for general practitioner principals in South East Scotland. *Educ Gen Pract* 1996; **7**: 249–54.

17 Burrows P, Millard L. Personal learning in general practice. *Educ Gen Pract* 1996; **7**: 300–5.

18 Gillies A. *The Clinician's Guide to Surviving IT*. Oxford: Radcliffe Publishing; 2006.

19 *The Cochrane Library.* www.library.nhs.uk

20 Brenner SH, McKinin EJ. CINAHL and MEDLINE: a comparison of indexing practices. *Bull Med Lib Assoc* 1989; **77**: 366–71.

21 Okuma E. Selecting CD-ROM databases for nursing students: a comparison of MEDLINE and the Cumulative Index to Nursing and Allied Health Literature (CINAHL). *Bull Med Lib Assoc* 1994; **82**: 25–9.

22 Watson MM, Perrin R. A comparison of CINAHL and MEDLINE CD-ROM in four allied health areas. *Bull Med Lib Assoc* 1994; **82**: 214–16.

23 Kiley R. Medical databases on the Internet – part 2. *J Roy Soc Med* 1997; **90**: 679–80.

24 Kiley R. How to get medical information from the Internet. *J Roy Soc Med* 1997; **90**: 488–90.

25 Kiley R. Evidence-based medicine on the Internet. *J Roy Soc Med* 1998; **91**: 74–5.

26 *Mentor Plus* is available from www.mentorplus.com/

27 Muir Gray JA. *Evidence-Based Healthcare.* 2nd ed. Edinburgh: Churchill Livingstone; 2001.

28 Carter Y, Howe A, Shaw S (eds). *Health Economics.* Master Classes in Primary Care Research No 9. London: Royal College of General Practitioners; 2005.

29 Kobelt G. *Health Economics: an introduction to economic evaluation.* 2nd ed. London: Office of Health Economics; 2002.

30 Tovey D (editorial director). *Clinical Evidence.* Issue 15. London: BMJ Publishing Group; 2006.

31 Kiley R. *The Doctor's Internet Handbook.* 2nd ed. London: Royal Society of Medicine; 2000.

32 Curtis HA, Lawrence CJ, Tripp JH. Teenage sexual intercourse and pregnancy. *Arch Dis Child* 1988; **63**: 373–9.

33 Francome C, Walsh J. *Young Teenage Pregnancy.* London: Middlesex University and Family Planning Association; 1995.

34 Pearson VAH, Owen MR, Phillips DR *et al.* Pregnant teenagers' knowledge and use of emergency contraception. *BMJ* 1995; **310**: 1644.

35 Greenhalgh T, Taylor R. How to read a paper: papers that go beyond numbers (qualitative research). *BMJ* 1997; **315**: 740–3.

36 Mays N, Pope C (eds). *Qualitative Research in Health Care.* 3rd ed. London: BMJ Publishing Group; 2006.

37 Murphy E, Dingwall R, Greatbatch D *et al.* Qualitative research methods in health technology assessment: a review of the literature. *Health Technol Assess* 1998; **2(16)**: 1–274.

38 Hannah M, Hannah W, Hewson S *et al.* Planned caesarean section versus planned vaginal birth for breech presentation at term: a randomised multicentre trial. *The Lancet* 2000; **357**: 1375–83.

39   Glezerman M. Five years to the term breech trial: the rise and fall of a randomised controlled trial. *American Journal of Obstetrics and Gynecology* 2006; **194**: 20–5.

40   Cronk M. Midwives and breech birth. *Practising Midwife* 1998; **1(7/8)**: 44–5.

41   Hogle KL, Kilburn L, Hewson S *et al.* Impact of the international term breech trial on clinical practice and concerns: a survey of centre collaborators. *J Obstet Gynaecol Can* 2003; **25**: 14–6.

42   Chambers R, Wakley G. *Making Clinical Governance Work for You.* Oxford: Radcliffe Medical Press; 2000.

43   Halligan A. *Clinical Governance – assuring the sacred duty of trust to patients.* Leicester: Clinical Governance Support Team; 2005.

44   Wakley G, Chambers R, Field S. *Continuing Professional Development: making it happen in primary care.* Oxford: Radcliffe Medical Press; 2000.

45   National Patient Safety Agency. *Seven Steps to Patient Safety. A guide for NHS staff.* London: NPSA; 2003.

46   Audit Commission. *Early Lessons in Implementing Practice Based Commissioning.* London: Audit Commission; 2006.

47   General Medical Council. *Management for Doctors.* London: General Medical Council; 2006.

48   Deegan M, Hensher M and colleagues on Local Hospitals Profit Board. *Strengthening Local Services: the future of the acute hospital.* London: National Leadership Network; 2006.

49   Dunning M, Abi-Aad G, Gilbert D *et al. Experience, Evidence and Everyday Practice.* London: King's Fund; 1999.

50   Taylor M. *Unleashing the Potential. Bringing residents to the centre of regeneration.* York: Joseph Rowntree Foundation; 1995.

51   Chambers R, Boath E, Drinkwater C. *Involving Patients and the Public: how to do it better.* 2nd ed. Oxford: Radcliffe Medical Press; 2003.

52   Department of Health. *The Caldicott Committee Report on the Review of Patient-identifiable Information.* London: Department of Health; 1997.

53   Donald P. Promoting local ownership of guidelines. *Guidelines in Practice* 2000; **3**: 17.

54   Department of Health. *Standards for Better Health.* London: Department of Health; 2004.

55   Cox J, King J, Hutchinson A, McAvoy P. *Understanding Doctors' Performance.* Oxford: Radcliffe Publishing; 2006.

56   Mohanna K, Chambers R. *Risk Matters in Healthcare.* Oxford: Radcliffe Medical Press; 2000. (Out of print)

57   Moore A, McQuay H. Statin safety: a perspective. *Bandolier* 2006; **13(5)**: 2–3.

58   Chambers R, Wakley G. *Clinical Audit in Primary Care. Demonstrating quality and outcomes.* Oxford: Radcliffe Publishing; 2005.

59   Lugon M, Singleton C. Chronic disease management and the implications for clinical governance. *Clinical Governance Bulletin* 2005; **6(2)**: 1–3.

60   Sheldon T, Cullum N, Dawson D *et al*. What's the evidence that NICE guidance has been implemented? Results from a national evaluation using time series analysis, audit of patients' notes, and interviews. *BMJ* 2004; **329**: 999–1004.

61   Chambers R, Wakley G, Blenkinsopp A. *Supporting Self-care in Primary Care*. Oxford: Radcliffe Publishing; 2006.

62   Healthcare Commission. *Annual Healthcheck*. London: Healthcare Commission; 2005. www.healthcarecommission.org.uk/annualhealthcheck

63   Wall D, Halligan A, Deighan M, Cullen R. Leadership, strategy and clinical governance. *Nexus Background* 2002; **4**: 1–7.

64   National Audit Office. *Achieving Improvements through Clinical Governance*. London: National Audit Office; 2003. www.nao.gov.uk/publications/nao_reports/02-03/02031055.pdf

65   James A. Making space for clinical governance. *ImpAct in Bandolier* 2000; **7(3)**: 5–6.

66   www.concordat.org.uk

67   Department of Health. *Research Governance Framework for Health and Social Care*. 2nd ed. London: Department of Health; 2005. www.dh.gov.uk

68   Department of Health. *The Regulation of the Non-medical Healthcare Professions: a review by the Department of Health*. London: Department of Health; 2006. www.dh.gov.uk/prod_consum_dh/groups/dh_digitalassets/@dh/@en/documents/digitalasset/dh_4137295.pdf

69   Secretary of State for Health. *Trust, Assurance and Safety. The Regulation of Health Professionals in the 21st Century*. London: The Stationery Office; 2007.

70   Chambers R, Tavabie A, Mohanna K *et al*. *The Good Appraisal Toolkit for Primary Care*. Oxford: Radcliffe Publishing; 2004.

71   Mason A, Chambers R, Conlon M *et al*. *Principles underlying the standards to be used in appraisal*. A series of papers commissioned by The Academy of Medical Royal Colleges of the Career Grade Doctor Appraisal Forum. www.appraisalsupport.nhs.uk

72   Home Secretary and Secretary of State for Health. *Learning from Tragedy, Keeping Patients Safe. Overview of the Government's action programme in response to the recommendations of the Shipman Inquiry*. London: DH; 2007.

73   Department of Health. *Building a Safer NHS for Patients: implementing 'an organisation with a memory'*. London: DH; 2001.

74   Grant J, Stanton F. *The Effectiveness of Continuing Professional Development*. Edinburgh: Association for the Study of Medical Education; 2000.

75   Mohanna K, Wall D, Chambers R. *Teaching Made Easy*. 2nd ed. Oxford: Radcliffe Medical Press; 2003.

76 Chambers R, Wakley G, Iqbal Z *et al. Prescription for Learning: techniques, games and activities*. Oxford: Radcliffe Medical Press; 2002.

77 Chambers R, editor. *A Guide to Accredited Professional Development. Preparing for revalidation*. London: Royal College of General Practitioners; 2002.

78 Chambers R, Wakley G. *Clinical Audit in Primary Care: demonstrating quality and outcomes*. Oxford: Radcliffe Publishing; 2005.

79 Chisholm A, Askham J. *What Do You Think of Your Doctor?* Oxford: Picker Institute Europe; 2006.

80 Howie JGR, Heaney D, Maxwell M *et al.* A comparison of the Patient Enablement Instrument (PEI) against two established satisfaction scales as an outcome measure of primary care consultations. *Family Practice* 1998; **15**: 165–71.

81 Marshall G, Hays R. *The Patient Satisfaction Questionnaire Short-Form (PSQ-18)*. Santa Monica, CA: RAND; 1994.

82 Picker Institute Europe. *Making Patients' Views Count*. Oxford: Picker Institute Europe; 2006. www.pickereurope.org

83 Chisholm A, Cairncross L, Askham J. *Setting Standards. The views of members of the public and doctors on the standards of care and practice they expect of doctors*. Oxford: Picker Institute Europe; 2006.

84 General Medical Council. *Good Medical Practice*. London: GMC; 2006. www.gmc-uk.org/guidance/good_medical_practice/GMC_GMP_V41.pdf

85 Eraut M, du Boulay B. *Developing the Attributes of Medical Professional Judgement and Competence*. Sussex: University of Sussex; 2000. www.informatics.sussex.ac.uk/users/bend/doh/

86 Royal College of General Practitioners and Brook. *Confidentiality and Young People. A toolkit for general practice, primary care groups and trusts*. London: Royal College of General Practitioners; 2000.

INDEX